INTERVENTIONAL
RADIOLOGY
explained

Published by ReMEDICA Publishing Limited
32-38 Osnaburgh Street, London, NW1 3ND, UK

Tel: +44 207 388 7677
Fax: +44 207 388 7678
Email: books@remedica.com
www.remedica.com

ReMEDICA Specialty Guides for Clinicians & GPs
ISSN 1472-4138; Volume 1
ISBN 1 901346 02 1
British Library Cataloguing-in-Publication Data
A catalogue record for this book is available from the British Library.

INTERVENTIONAL RADIOLOGY
explained

I S Francis, FRCS, MBBS, BDS (Hons)
A F Watkinson, FRCS, FRCR

Department of Radiology
The Royal Free Hospital, London, UK

ReMEDICAPUBLISHING

ACKNOWLEDGEMENTS

We would like to express appreciation to our colleagues, who perform many of the procedures described in this book on a day to day basis. We would especially like to acknowledge the role of the radiographers, in particular Scott Martin, at the Royal Free Hospital, who was instrumental in formatting and compiling many of the patient information sheets.

Finally, thanks to all at ReMEDICA for their support throughout this project.

ISF
AFW

FOREWORD

This book fills a much needed gap by providing a clear, informative, easy to read guide to interventional radiology. Such has been the speed of growth in this area in the last few years that most clinicians and general practitioners will acknowledge gaps in their knowledge which this well written text will fill. The format is reader friendly and this would be an excellent book to have on a ward, in the doctor's office or on the shelves at home.

Each section not only describes an interventional technique and its expected outcome but also gives a succinct description of presentation, investigation and treatment options. The patient section is equally useful and something which has long been needed. It is so easy for a doctor to believe that they have adequately explained a technique to a patient. This is often not the case and the patient section enhances the book. Information sheets provided in this book should be copied and kept in the out patients department and on the wards. There will certainly be refinements and expansion of interventional techniques in the next few years and I hope the authors are already thinking about their second edition.

Carol M Black MD FRCP F Med Sci
Professor of Rheumatology
Royal Free Campus
London, UK

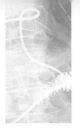

CONTENTS

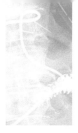

INTRODUCTION

Interventional radiology is a relatively new specialty, having evolved rapidly in the last 30 years. This has been fueled by the explosive growth of real time imaging and technological advances in the design of guide wires, catheters and balloons. These developments continue at pace and it is difficult enough for those working within this sub-specialty of radiology to keep up to date with the changes.

Our goal in this book is to provide clear information on the indications, techniques and outcomes of the full spectrum of interventional procedures, in a format that we hope will appeal to general radiologists, clinicians and general practitioners alike. To assist with patient understanding of interventional procedures, all the techniques have a specifically designed patient information form. Please copy this and distribute to your patients.

We hope that you find this book both informative and stimulating, and that it serves to provide an insight into the exciting and rapidly changing world of interventional radiology.

GENERAL INTERVENTIONAL RADIOLOGY

1.1 Informed Consent

Interventional radiology involves a high degree of patient contact and the regular use of invasive technical procedures. Consequently, it is important to establish a good radiologist/patient relationship and to obtain informed consent before embarking upon any procedure.

As with all invasive procedures, some general guidelines should be followed:

- The procedure should be undertaken only if there is a clear clinical indication
- Any procedure should be in the best interest of the patient
- The potential benefits of the procedure should outweigh the risks

The patient usually remains under the joint care of the referring clinician and the radiologist. As such, it is essential that, prior to any invasive procedure, there is open dialogue between the clinician and the radiologist. This should allow the establishment of the indications and implications for the therapy, as well as general agreement as to the appropriateness of the proposed treatment. To this end, the referring clinician should be aware of the nature of the procedure to be undertaken, the likely outcome and all possible complications.

Ultimately, it should be the interventional radiologist who explains the procedure and obtains the informed consent. Ideally this should be undertaken away from the interventional suite, so that full and detailed discussion can take place and the patient can be free to question and digest the information. During this dialogue, the patient should be informed of any common or significant risks associated with the procedure, the details of which vary between clinicians and the systems in which they practise.

The use of sound clinical practice and the establishment of a good rapport with both the patient and the referring clinician will result in improved patient co-operation and clinical colleagues will have a better regard for the limitations of the techniques used. These factors together with careful attention to detail will minimise possible litigation resulting from procedures undertaken by the interventional radiologist.

It is important that appropriate clinical back-up (anaesthetic, surgical, nursing) is sought before embarking on an interventional procedure. Adequate patient analgesia and sedation should be available, along with appropriate monitoring. Accurate note-keeping is essential, and any difficulties or problems encountered should be fully documented. Clear guidelines for follow-up of the patient – both while the individual remains an inpatient and subsequently following discharge – should be established.

1.2 Analgesia and Sedation

Interventional techniques require patient co-operation. In order to achieve this, the patient must be comfortable and pain free. Although a small amount of interventional radiology is undertaken under general anaesthesia, the vast majority of work involves the use of sedation and analgesic techniques.

At the extremes of age or in the extremely sick patient, operators should have a low threshold for requesting anaesthetic assistance. This enables safe analgesia and sedation to be given, ensuring that the interventional radiologist can concentrate on the technical details of the procedure.

Analgesics

Enable adequate pain control

Lignocaine

Most commonly used analgesic
Used as 1% plain solution/2.5% with adrenaline (1:200 000)
Maximum single dose for a 70 kg patient is 200 mg (20 ml of 1% lignocaine)

Opioid analgesics

Relieve moderate to severe pain by acting on specific receptors, although they have dose-related side effects that result in respiratory depression and hypotension
Administered by slow intravenous injection; the quantity is titrated against the continuing pain and the associated side effects

Sedation

Oral premedication

Diazepam and temazepam are effective oral sedatives that are used prior to the start of an interventional procedure (Figure 1.21)
Diazepam is normally given the night before whereas temazepam is given 1 h prior to the procedure.

Figure 1.21
Vials of local anaesthetic (lignocaine), sedative (midazolam) and analgesic (pethidine)

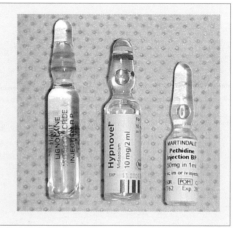

Diazepam	Temazepam	
Adult	15 mg in divided doses	10–20 mg
Children	10 mg (if less than 3 years, 5 mg)	1 mg per kg

Table 1.21 Recommended doses of diazepam and temazepam for oral premedication

Intravenous sedation

Midazolam is the benzodiazepine recommended by the RCS (Royal College of Surgeons) Working Party on Sedation for Non-Anaesthetists; as such, it is widely used in interventional radiological procedures

Before using an intravenous sedative, it is recommended that all staff are adequately trained in resuscitation techniques and facilities are available for both monitoring and recovery

All operator sedationists are advised to undergo resuscitation update/ACLS (Advanced Cardiac Life Support) training every 5 years and this is certainly what most departments aim for

The sedative is given in 2 mg aliquots until a satisfactory level of sedation is achieved – the patient should be responsive to commands but appear relaxed

Full monitoring is maintained throughout the sedation, and oxygen is given

Particular care must be taken when sedation is used in conjunction with opioids as their effects are synergistic

1.3 Interventional Suite Design

A radiology nurse receives patients undergoing an interventional procedure in the department. In the interventional suite the patient lies on the X-ray table on a mattress with a pillow for head support (Figure 1.31). Some suites have the facility to provide music of the patient's choice. Following the procedure the patients are looked after in a recovery suite or day ward by a radiology nurse familiar with X-ray guided procedures.

1.4 Percutaneous Biopsy and Drainage

Percutaneous approaches for biopsy and drainage have proved to be of great value in the management of an array of clinical problems and have almost replaced open surgical drainage procedures. These techniques are within the scope of all departments and are practised in most clinical centres. Provided the lesion can be imaged, percutaneous access can be achieved. The range of applications for these basic interventional procedures has evolved along with improved imaging modalities and percutaneous instruments.

Presentation

Radiologically detected abnormality requiring:

Biopsy

Avoidance of open procedure/general anaesthetic
Allows the establishment of histological/cytological diagnosis

Drainage

Accurate localization and safe drainage using standard angiographic techniques (Seldinger – see appendix)
Allows continual drainage using a locking pigtail catheter
Allows microbiological analysis, so improving targeting with appropriate chemotherapy
In sites of chronic infection (empyema), allows local thrombolysis, so improving clinical outcome
Avoidance of open procedure/general anaesthetic

Contraindications

Absolute

None

Relative

Abnormal coagulation profile (platelets <50 000; INR >1.5)
Hypervascular lesion
Immunosuppression
Poor patient co-operation

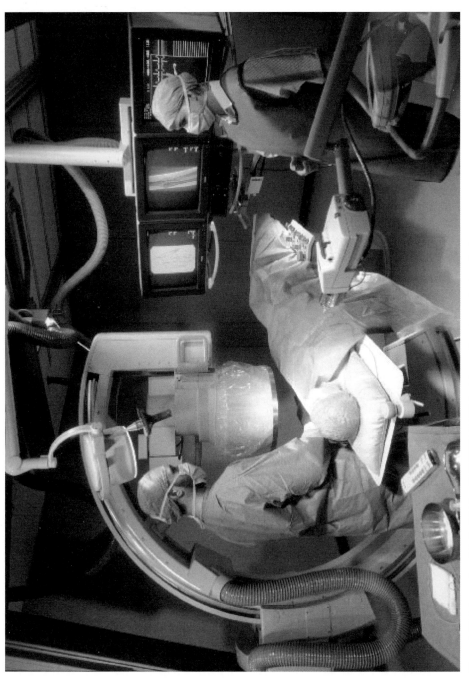

Figure 1.31 Interventional Suite (Philips INTEGRIS V5000 for interventional vascular imaging)

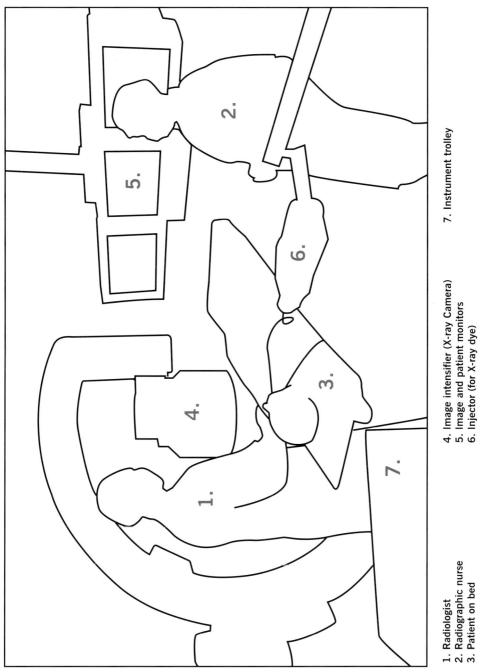

1. Radiologist
2. Radiographic nurse
3. Patient on bed

4. Image intensifier (X-ray Camera)
5. Image and patient monitors
6. Injector (for X-ray dye)

7. Instrument trolley

| **Investigations** | Routine blood screens |
| | Appropriate imaging to evaluate the lesion to be biopsied or the site to be drained (Figure 1.41, 1.42) |

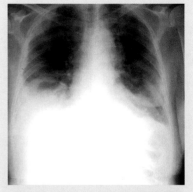

Figure 1.41
Erect chest X-ray of a post-operative patient with a right pleural effusion

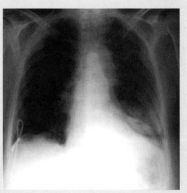

Figure 1.42
A pigtail catheter in situ and complete resolution of the effusion

Treatment options

Surgical

Open biopsy/drainage

Associated with increased morbidity/mortality

Interventional therapy

Can be carried out under any modality, providing the lesion can be visualized – depends upon local availability and personal preference

	Ultrasound	Fluoroscopy	CT	MRI
Advantages	Real time	Widely available	Good localization	Real time
	Portable	Biplanar imaging	Excellent visualization of surrounding structures	Does not use ionizing radiation
	Does not use ionizing radiation	Improves localization		
	Cheap			
Disadvantages	Patient and operator dependent	Interposed structures not visible	Increased procedural time	Not readily available
	Makes accurate targeting of deep seated lesions difficult	Lesion may not be visible under fluoroscopy	Expensive	Requires special equipment
			Involves high-dose ionizing radiation	Long procedural time
				Expensive

Table 1.41 Advantages and disadvantages of various guidance techniques

Patient preparation

Informed consent

Local anaesthetic ± sedation

(Figure 1.43, 1.44)

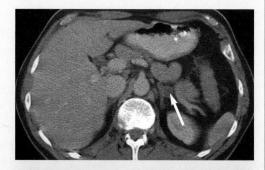

Figure 1.43
Supine CT scan illustrating an enlarged left adrenal gland

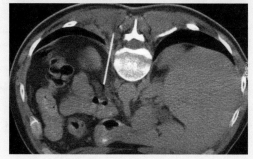

Figure 1.44
Prone CT guided biopsy of left adrenal gland

1. Biopsy	Wide choice of needles available – vary from small gauge, which allow aspiration, to large-gauge core biopsy
	Type of needle depends upon both the site and the nature of the specimen being biopsied
	Increase in needle size increases the chances of a positive yield but also results in increased complications
Procedure	Under aseptic technique, the lesion is identified using the most appropriate imaging modality
	It is essential to:
	• position the needle accurately
	• sample different parts of the lesion
	• perform multiple passes
Outcome	Good technical success, with a high positive yield, and can easily be repeated
	Fine-needle aspiration outcomes are very dependent upon local cytological services
Complications	Haematoma formation
	Infection
	Damage to adjacent structures
2. Drainage	Techniques used are the same as for biopsy
	All imaging modalities can be used
	Avoidance of the transgression of vital structures is obviously vital, but, where possible, the shortest route is generally chosen (Figures 1.45–1.48)
Procedure	A needle puncture is performed and a guidewire advanced into the site for drainage (Seldinger technique – see appendix) – this allows safe access to the cavity to be drained
	Once access is secured, the tract is dilated and a locking pigtail catheter inserted
	A sample of fluid is sent for microbiological analysis and the catheter is left on free drainage

Outcome	Excellent results
Complications	As for biopsy

Figure 1.45
CT scan with patient prone. Large left psoas abscess. Skin markers in place

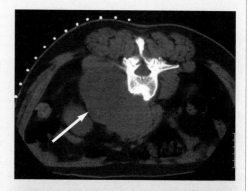

Figure 1.46
Abscess localized and tract infiltrated with local anaesthetic

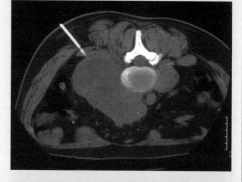

Figure 1.47
Drain introduced into abscess cavity

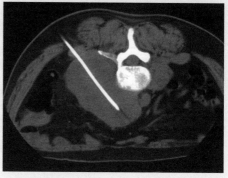

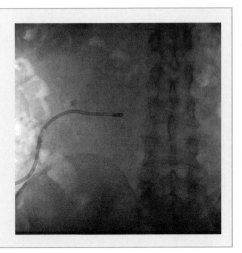

Figure 1.48
Locking pigtail trail within
right psoas collection

1.5 Stent Design

A stent is a form of scaffolding used to contain and reinforce the patency of a biological conduit. The addition of stents to the armamentarium of the interventional radiologist has been dramatic. Their rapid development has resulted in ever-increasing indications for their use. Stents are now routinely used in the vascular and biliary systems, the gastrointestinal and urinary tracts, and the tracheobronchial system (Figure 1.51, 1.52).

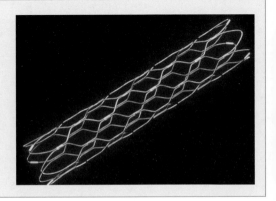

Figure 1.51
Nickel-titanium alloy
vascular stent

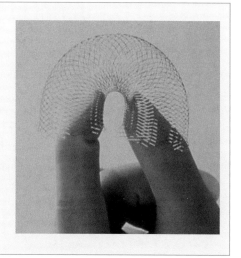

Figure 1.52
Stainless steel
gastrointestinal stent

Stents can be constructed of plastic or metal.

Plastic stents are mainly used in the hepatobiliary or the urinary system. They are constructed so as to allow their removal and replacement when necessary.

Metal stents come in two basic forms:

* Balloon expandable – these are passively expanded by a balloon system; once the balloon has been deflated, they do not expand any further
* Self-expanding – conversely, these have an inherent capacity to expand based on a thermal memory

Metal stents are made of stainless steel, tantalum and nitinol (nickel-titanium alloy).

Although stents are very successful, they still have associated problems. These include occlusion with thrombus or tumour and intimal hyperplasia. It is in these areas that active research continues and that the next advances are awaited.

ULTRASOUND BIOPSY/ASPIRATION

What is a biopsy? This is the removal of a small amount of tissue from the body. This is then examined under a microscope to establish a diagnosis.

What is an aspiration? This is the removal of fluid from an area of the body, e.g. fluid in a cyst, abscess or collection.

Preparation You may be admitted to a hospital bed or attend as a day case. You will be asked to sign a consent form.

What happens? The area to be examined is identified using ultrasound.

Biopsy – the area is cleaned and a local anaesthetic is used to numb the skin. A needle is inserted into the area and some tissue is withdrawn. Ultrasound allows accurate 'targeting' of the site of interest.

Aspiration – the area is cleaned and a local anaesthetic is used to numb the skin. A small needle is inserted into the area being examined and fluid is withdrawn through the needle.

How long will it take? Usually up to 30 minutes.

Afterwards The aftercare depends on the type of biopsy being performed. This will be explained to you at the time of the examination.

Results The sample of tissue/fluid is sent for analysis. Your doctor will be contacted with the results. This can take up to 3 days.

COMPUTED TOMOGRAPHY (CT) GUIDED BIOPSY/ASPIRATION

What is a CT guided biopsy/aspiration?

A biopsy is a procedure in which a sample of tissue is taken from you so it can be tested to determine its nature.

An aspiration is a procedure whereby fluid is removed from you so it can be tested to determine its nature. To avoid you having an operation it is possible to take these samples with a fine needle. A radiologist uses CT to position the needle accurately.

Preparation

The exact nature of the procedure will be unique to you and so an explanation will be given to you by the radiologist. You will have to sign a consent form to show you have understood the explanation.

What happens?

Usually an inpatient procedure but can be a day case. You will have a CT scan to locate the affected area. The skin surface will be marked above this area. The radiologist will clean the skin with antiseptic then 'freeze' the area with local anaesthetic. This will sting at first and then go numb. From then on you will only feel pushing as the radiologist positions the needle. When in position you will be scanned to ensure the needle is in the correct location and the sample will be taken. If you are having fluid drained the radiologist may find it necessary to put a small tube (drain) in so the fluid can continue draining after the procedure is over. Finally a small dressing is applied.

Afterwards

You will be monitored for a short time after the procedure to ensure there is no bleeding. When the local anaesthetic wears off you may feel slightly sore over the needle site.

If you had a chest biopsy/aspiration you will need a chest X-ray after 4 hours. There is a slight chance air may be introduced between your lung and your chest wall causing your lung to collapse, and making you short of breath. Your doctor can then take steps to re-inflate your lung.

Results

After the sample has been analyzed the results will be sent to your hospital doctor and GP, who will then discuss them with you.

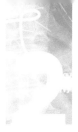

GASTROINTESTINAL INTERVENTION

2.1 Enteral Feeding

Traditionally enteral feeding was achieved either by direct surgical access or in the case of gastrostomies via percutaneous endoscopic routes (PEGs). This technique, as well as gastrojejunostomies (PGJ), can now be performed by interventional radiologists. These percutaneous techniques are associated with high technical success and low morbidity.

Indications

To allow enteral nutrition in cases of neurological, neoplastic and psychiatric disease
Malabsorption or small bowel disease
Where long term nutritional support is required
Prophylactically in patients requiring caloric build up prior to major surgery

Contraindications

Absolute

The presence of interposed bowel between the stomach and the anterior abdominal wall (transverse colon), when using the percutaneous route

Relative

Previous gastric surgery
Hepatomegaly
Ascites
Coagulopathy

Interventional therapy

Patient preparation

Informed consent

Intravenous access

Local anaesthetic + sedation +/– analgesia (opioid)

NG tube placement

Cessation of feeding for six hours prior to the procedure

Procedure

The left lobe of the liver is localized by ultrasound

Gaseous distension of the stomach is performed via an NG tube or following placement of an angiographic catheter if there is disease of the distal oesophagus (Figure 2.11, 2.12)

Fluoroscopy (lateral screening) is used to confirm that there is no interposing bowel or left lobe of liver between the stomach and the anterior abdominal wall

Apposition of the stomach wall and anterior abdominal wall is maintained throughout the procedure using retention devices introduced via needle puncture

A standard angiographic puncture is performed and a guidewire passed through the pylorus of the stomach into the jejunum (Figure 2.13, 2.14)

Serial dilatation is performed and the feeding tube advanced over the guidewire either into the stomach (Figure 2.15) or in the case of jejunostomies to just beyond the DJ flexure (Figure 2.16). Confirmation of the position of the tube is verified using contrast medium (Figure 2.17). The catheter is then fixed in place either by a suture or a fixation device (Figure 2.18).

Figure 2.11
Control film with NG tube
in stomach

Figure 2.12
NG tube within stomach.
Angiographic puncture

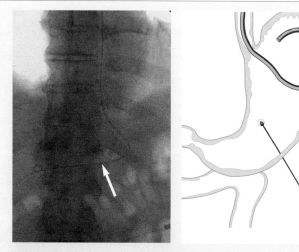

Figure 2.13
Angiographic puncture
with confirmation of entry
within stomach lumen

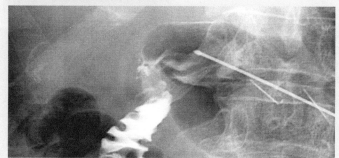

Figure 2.14
Guidewire advanced over
angiographic catheter into
the duodenum

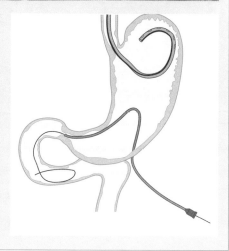

Figure 2.15
Guidewire advanced
through pylorus to level of
DJ flexure

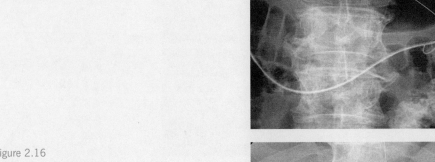

Figure 2.16
Following serial dilatation
feeding tube advanced over
guidewire into position

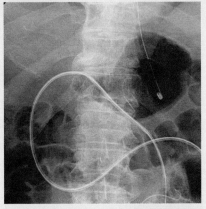

Figure 2.17
Contrast introduced via
jejunostomy tube to
confirm position. Retention
loop formed within
stomach

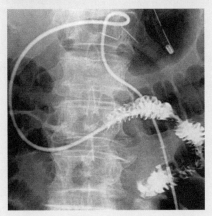

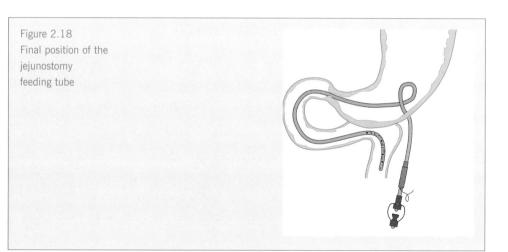

Figure 2.18
Final position of the
jejunostomy
feeding tube

Post-procedurally the patient is kept nil by mouth for 24 hours and
regular cardiovascular observations are undertaken. Feeding regime
is then commenced the following day.

The feeding tube should be routinely changed every 4-6 months.
This is easily performed on an outpatient basis once a tract is
established.

Outcome

High technical success rate in excess of 98% for gastrostomies, and
approximately 93% for jejunostomies

Complications

Major: (1.4%) – aspiration, peritonitis, haemorrhage

Minor: (2.9%) – peritonism, infection

**Gastrostomy vs.
jejunostomy**

There continues to be active debate as to which type of feeding
tube should be used. Gastrostomy tube placement is associated
with increased risk of aspiration. Percutaneous jejunostomies,
although requiring more procedural time and a small increase in
technical difficulty, markedly reduce the risk of gastroesophageal
reflux and aspiration and remain the best option in bed bound
supine patients or those with neurological deficits.

2.2 Enteric Strictures

Pathological narrowing of the bowel lumen can occur at any point
throughout the gastrointestinal system

Causes can be subdivided into intrinsic and extrinsic

Genetic	Malrotation
	Ladds' bands
Inflammatory	Peptic
	Inflammatory bowel disease
	Diverticular disease
Post-surgical	Anastomotic narrowing
	Adhesion
Neoplastic	Primary
	Secondary

Table 2.21 Causes of bowel strictures

Traditionally, interventional techniques were reserved for
oesophageal pathologies, but all enteric strictures are now
within the scope of the interventional radiologist

Strictures can be accessed via either an oral, rectal or stomal approach

Figure 2.22
Interventional stenting of
enteric strictures

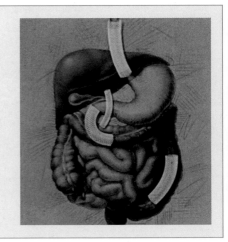

2.3 Oesophageal Strictures

Presentation

Dysphagia, weight loss, regurgitation
The duration of the history gives a further idea of the exact nature of the stricture

Investigations

Barium swallow
Upper gastrointestinal endoscopy + biopsy/brushings
Staging with ultrasound/CT if the stricture is of a malignant nature

Treatment options

Endoscopic dilation ± stenting
Surgical resection
Lasering

Treatment choice is dependent upon the nature and aetiology of the stricture and local expertise

Interventional therapy

Patient preparation

Informed consent
Intravenous access
Sedation
Antibiotic cover
Fast for 6 h prior to the procedure

1. Balloon Dilatation

Procedure

The stricture is outlined using water-soluble contrast medium (Figure 2.31)
This is then traversed using a standard guidewire and steerable catheter
Care should be taken with malignant strictures as there is an increased risk of guidewire perforation
Stricture treatment can take the form of balloon dilatation either with or without stent placement
Benign strictures are almost universally treated with balloon dilatation alone, whilst malignant strictures may benefit from

stent placement

Balloon size is based on the dimensions of the adjacent normal oesophagus

Figure 2.31
Contrast swallow demonstrating a dilated oesophagus with food debris within the lumen. At the gastroesophageal junction there is a smooth beak-like taper. These findings are typical of achalasia

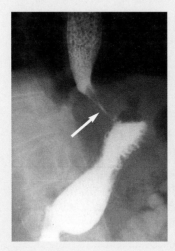
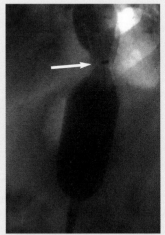

Figure 2.32
The distal oesophageal narrowing has been traversed and balloon dilatation is being performed. Note the 'waisting' of the balloon at the level of the stenosis

Figure 2.33
Post dilatation contrast swallow shows considerable improvement with no evidence of any leak

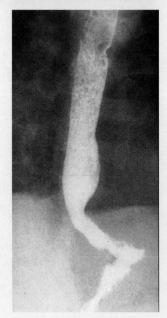

The balloon is inflated until the radiological 'waist' is eliminated (Figure 2.32)

Pressures should be kept less than 6 atmospheres otherwise the risk of perforation/spontaneous rupture increases

This treatment can be repeated on several occasions if required

Post-dilatation, a contrast examination is performed to ensure there is no evidence of mucosal tear or perforation (Figure 2.33)

If a tear or perforation is visualized, conservative management (nil by mouth, NG tube placement, intravenous antibiotics) will usually suffice. In malignant perforation a covered stent may be appropriate

Post-procedurally, the patient is kept under observation for 4 h, after which time, if there are no complications, normal diet can be resumed

Outcome

High technical success rate depending upon the nature of the stricture

Recurrence rate for caustic strictures is approximately 30% at 2 years

Poor outcome for malignant strictures treated with balloon dilatation alone – the majority of patients show recurrence of symptoms after a short period of time (days/weeks)

2. Stenting

The use of expandable metallic prostheses within the oesophagus is still primarily reserved for exophytic mural malignant lesions

Stents in benign disease are only used in exceptional circumstances

Although some stent designs now allow stent removal within a fixed time period, the indications for stent deployment in benign disease remain limited

There are currently a wide number of oesophageal stents available, including covered and uncovered, self-expanding and balloon expandable

Figure 2.34
Unenhanced CT scan
showing circumferential
thickening of the distal
oesophagus (arrow)

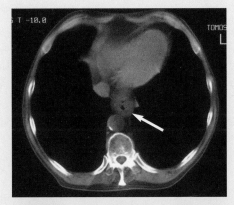

Figure 2.35
Barium swallow confirms
an irregular stricture of
the distal oesophagus.
Histology proved the
lesion to be a squamous
cell carcinoma

Figure 2.36
A Wallstent has been
placed across the
stricture. There is now
rapid flow of barium into
the stomach

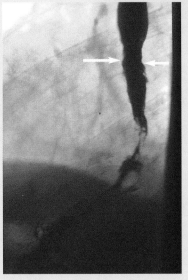
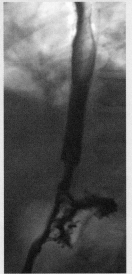

Procedure

The stricture is visualized using non-ionic contrast medium
(Figure 2.34, 2.35)

A standard catheter guidewire technique is then used to traverse
the stenosis/occlusion

The upper and lower limits of the lesion can be demonstrated and
a suitably sized prosthesis can be chosen to cover the entire length
of the stricture

The stent is deployed under fluoroscopic guidance – accurate positioning is essential to ensure the stricture is crossed in its entirety and to prevent distal migration (Figure 2.36)

Balloon dilatation can be performed before or after stent deployment depending upon the type of stent used

Post-procedurally, the patient is monitored closely for 4 h, after which time clear fluids are allowed

The following day, a repeat swallow examination should be performed. If there is no evidence of any leak, and free flow of contrast is seen into the stomach, the patient may resume a soft diet

If a perforation or a leak is demonstrated, the patient should be kept nil by mouth, given intravenous antibiotics and H_2 blockers; they should be placed on a course of total parenteral nutrition until such time as a swallow demonstrates closure of the perforation or leak

If at the time of the swallow there is early distal migration of the oesophageal stent, a second overlapping stent can be used to prevent further dislodgement

Outcome

Technical success rate is approximately 100%, with successful palliation being seen in approximately 80% of patients

Complications

Gastroesophageal reflux (0–20%)
Food impaction (5–10%)
Stent migration (0–30%, although less with modern stent designs)
Tumour overgrowth/ingrowth (5–30%) – this is obviously not a problem with covered stents, but this advantage has to be balanced against the fact that covered stents have a higher rate of distal migration (10–25%); modern stent designs have reduced this incidence

Stent-related mortality – upper gastrointestinal
haemorrhage/aspiration pneumonia (0–60%)

2.4 Gastric Outlet Obstruction

Presentation

History of recurrent non-bilious vomiting
Clinically, patients may exhibit the classical 'succussion splash'
Outlet obstruction occurs secondary to gastroparesis, chronic
paralytic ileus, post-operative strictures, peptic disease, malignant
disease or caustic ingestion

Investigations

Plain abdominal X-ray
Barium meal and follow-through
Endoscopy
CT (Figure 2.41)

These tests allow the confirmation of the underlying cause for
the gastric outlet obstruction and the establishment of a formal
treatment plan

Figure 2.41
CT showing pyloric
tumour mass extending
into 2nd part of
duodenum (arrow)

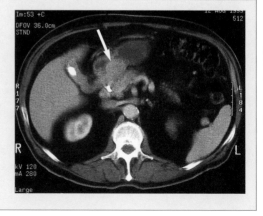

Treatment options

Medical management

For patients with benign peptic disease, proton-pump inhibitors and H_2 antagonists have become standard practice and have markedly changed the outcome in this group of individuals

Surgery

Surgical resection or drainage via a gastroenterostomy remains the mainstay of treatment in those patients with outlet obstruction who fail to respond to medical treatment or are obstructed due to malignant disease; however, balloon dilatation and stent placement are increasingly being performed

Interventional therapy

Patient preparation

Informed consent
Intravenous access
Local anaesthetic $\pm$ sedation
Nil by mouth for 6 h prior to the procedure

1. Balloon dilatation

Used for those patients with benign disease in whom surgery is contraindicated

Procedure

Using fluoroscopic guidance, the pyloric or anastomotic stricture is crossed using a combination of a trackable guidewire and steerable angiographic catheter

Contrast injection is used to visualize and size the stricture
This is then dilated using a balloon over a stiff guidewire, to a maximum diameter of 15–20 mm
Post-dilatation contrast examination is performed to rule out perforation
Post-procedurally, the patient is kept nil by mouth for 4 h and regular observations are carried out; after this period, if there are no complications, normal diet can be recommended

Outcome	Significant rate of failed cannulation (30%), especially in patients with large stomachs or gastrojejunostomies. Endoscopic assistance may increase success rate of stricture cannulation
	Long-term success – approximately 70% at 2-year follow-up
Complications	Mucosal tear/perforation

2. Stenting

Is evolving as a therapeutic option in upper gastrointestinal pathology, mainly in malignant strictures, where other treatment options are not feasible

Recently, licensing of gastrointestinal stents has been granted for gastric outlet obstruction and duodenal strictures

The technique is similar to that used for balloon dilatation, except the stent is placed before the stricture is dilated

(Figures 2.42–2.44)

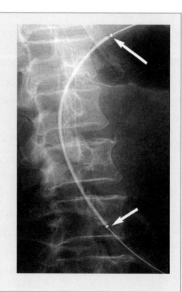

Figure 2.42
Stricture crossed with guidewire and stent prior to release

Figure 2.43
Stent released into final
position extending from
pylorus to junction of 2nd
and 3rd part of duodenum
(biliary metal stent also
present)

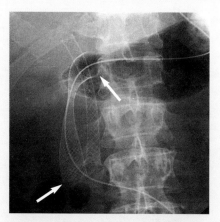

Figure 2.44
Contrast study
demonstrating free flow of
contrast through stent into
distal duodenum

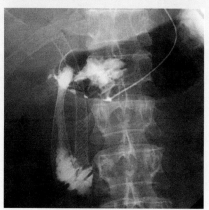

No information is currently available for the long-term patency
of these stents and they are presently only indicated for
advanced malignant disease in patients not fit to undergo
operative intervention

2.5 Colonic Strictures

Causes can be inflammatory, post-surgical or neoplastic in nature.
Until recently, interventional therapy was restricted to balloon
dilatation of anastomotic strictures; however, recent developments
in stent design have resulted in the stenting of malignant colonic

strictures in patients. There are currently two main indications for the use of colonic stents.

1. Acute presentation – stenting to allow improved clinical condition and full staging followed by tumour resection and primary anastomoses rather than emergency operation and defunctioning colostomy followed by second stage procedure to resect the bowel tumour

2. Palliation – the stenting of inoperable malignant strictures in patients unfit for any other form of palliation

Presentation

Symptoms of large-bowel obstruction, with complete constipation, abdominal distension and late onset vomiting

Procedure

The patient is placed in a standard left lateral decubitus position
A barium enema tube is introduced into the rectum, and the stricture is visualized using a water-soluble contrast medium (Figure 2.51)
A standard guidewire and steerable catheter is then used to cross the stricture

Interventional therapy

Patient preparation

Informed consent
Intravenous access - sedation
Antibiotic cover

Bowel preparation is not usually feasible because the patients are completely obstructed, although a phosphate enema may be given prior to the procedure

1. Balloon dilatation

Normally indicated in benign disease, not malignant due to risk of perforation

Balloons of up to 40 mm in diameter can be used within the rectosigmoid region

The disappearance of radiological waisting denotes the success of the procedure

A persistent waist in a setting of adequate balloon pressures dictates that the procedure should be abandoned, in order to avoid possible perforation or tearing

Following dilatation, a contrast study should be performed to confirm the absence of any local complications

Post-procedurally, the patient should be kept on close observation for 4 h, monitoring for signs of peritonitis, after which time a normal diet can be resumed

Outcome

Technical success varies depending upon the exact site and nature of the stricture

A combination of radiological and endoscopic techniques has been used in the past for proximal lesions

Complications

Perforation

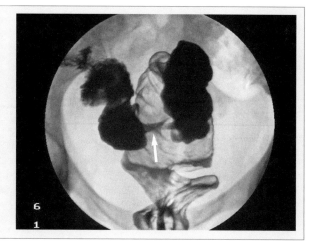

Figure 2.51
Double contrast enema showing a short extrinsic stricture within the sigmoid colon (arrow). Patient known to have disseminated malignancy (Posterior - Anterior view)

2. Stenting

Self-expanding stents are deployed in the colon
Their deployment is achieved by a standard catheter guidewire
technique, following visualization of the stricture (Figure 2.52, 2.53)

Outcome

Combined interventional-endoscopic approaches are sometimes
necessary for proximal large bowel strictures
No large series results have yet been published

Complications

Perforation

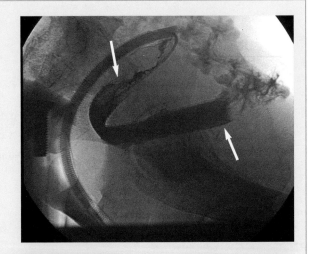

Figure 2.52
Stricture crossed and a
colonic stent in position
(arrows). Free flow of
contrast demonstrated
(Lateral view)

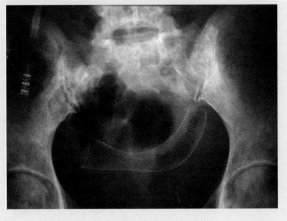

Figure 2.53
Final position of colonic
stent. Multiple metastatic
bony deposits noted
(Anterior - Posterior view)

RADIOLOGICALLY INSERTED FEEDING TUBE

What is a feeding tube?

Your doctors feel that you are not taking sufficient food by mouth to get fit and well. In order to build you up, a small feeding tube will be placed directly in your stomach.

How long will it take?

The approximate time for this procedure is 45 minutes.

Is it painful?

You will be given oxygen and you can have a sedative injection via a vein in your hand. This will make you sleepy, but will still allow you to co-operate during the procedure.

What happens?

In the X-ray department you will be expected to lie flat on your back on an X-ray table. A tube will be passed through your nose into your stomach to allow it to be inflated with air. A local anaesthetic injection will be given into the front of your abdomen. The feeding tube will be passed into your stomach via the abdominal wall under X-ray control. It will then be fixed in place with a plastic disc or suture.

Afterwards

You will not be able to start using the feeding tube for 24 h post procedure. During this time you will be kept on a drip.

Whilst in hospital you will be taught how to look after the feeding tube, and a feeding regimen to meet your dietary needs will be established.

It is important never to put very thick liquids or poorly crushed tablets down the tube. After each use, the tube should be flushed with water.

If the tube does become blocked, immediately inform your GP or district nurse so that they can contact the radiology department. The tube is routinely changed every 4-6 months.

The district nurse normally does this.

OESOPHAGEAL DILATATION/ STENTING

What is oesophageal dilatation/stenting?

If the oesophagus has become blocked or narrowed and prevents a person from normal eating and drinking, it can be widened using an X-ray procedure.

Preparation

The nurses on the ward will help to get you ready. You must not eat for 4 h before the procedure and a doctor on the ward will explain the procedure to you so that you can sign a consent form. Please ask any questions you wish.

What happens?

You will be asked to lie on your front on the X-ray table. The throat is sprayed with a local anaesthetic, and a small tube is passed down the oesophagus until it has crossed the narrowing or blockage. A small balloon, which is attached to the end of the tube, is then expanded. This in turn widens the oesophagus. This is performed a number of times with different sized balloons until the narrowing has disappeared. Under special circumstances, a metallic stent (spring) is then put in place to stop the narrowing returning.

Is it painful?

The back of the throat is sprayed with local anaesthetic before the procedure so that the throat is numbed and the tube cannot be felt going in and out. The procedure can be uncomfortable and therefore sedation and painkillers are given if required.

How long does it take?

The procedure will usually be completed within an hour and you will have to lie on your front for this period.

Afterwards

When the procedure is finished you must stay in bed for a couple of hours or until the sedation wears off. You should not eat anything for 4 h post-procedure and a nurse will take regular checks of your pulse and blood pressure. If you experience any pain after the dilatation, tell the nurse looking after you, who will give you some painkillers.

Results

A doctor on the ward will talk to you about the procedure shortly after it. A copy of the test results will be sent to your GP.

If a stent ('spring') has been placed across the narrowing, the next morning you may return to the X-ray department for a check X-ray. Your diet will need to continue to be modified such that bulky foods – especially cuts of meat – are avoided. Regular fluids should be taken. Carbonated drinks are advised to keep the stent patent.

GASTRIC OUTLET OBSTRUCTION

What is gastric outlet balloon dilatation and stenting?

This is a procedure using X-rays, to widen the outlet to the stomach or duodenum, that is the part of the intestine leading out of the stomach. This is necessary, if it has become blocked or narrowed and prevents a person from normal eating and drinking.

Preparation

The nurses on the ward will help to get you ready. You must not eat for 4 h before the procedure and a doctor on the ward will explain the procedure to you so that you can sign a consent form. Please ask any questions you wish.

What happens?

You will be asked to lie on your back on the X-ray table.
The throat is sprayed with a local anaesthetic and a small tube is passed down the oesophagus and through into the stomach, until it has crossed the narrowing or blockage. A small balloon, which is attached to the end of the tube, is then expanded. This in turn dilates the duodenum. This is performed a number of times until the narrowing has disappeared. Under special circumstances, a metallic stent is then put in place to stop the narrowing returning (usually if the underlying cause is malignant).

Is it painful?

The back of the throat is sprayed with local anaesthetic before the procedure so that the throat is numbed and the tube cannot be felt going in and out. The procedure can be uncomfortable and therefore sedation and painkillers are given if required.

How long will it take?

The procedure will usually be completed within an hour and you will have to lie on your back for this period.

Afterwards

When the procedure is finished you must stay in bed for a couple of hours or until the sedation wears off. You should not eat anything for 4 h post procedure and a nurse will take regular checks of your pulse and blood pressure. If you experience any pain after the dilatation, tell the nurse looking after you, who will give you some painkillers.

Results

A doctor on the ward will talk to you about the procedure shortly after it. A copy of the test results will be sent to your GP.
If a stent ('spring') has been placed across the narrowing, the next morning you will return to the X-ray department for a check X-ray. Your diet will need to continue to be modified such that bulky foods – especially cuts of meat – are avoided. Regular fluids should be taken. Carbonated drinks are advised.

COLONIC STENTING

What is colonic stenting?

This is a procedure to widen the colon, that is the part of the intestine lying in the pelvis. This is necessary if it has become blocked or narrowed preventing you from passing normal motions and an operation is not advisable.

Preparation

The nurses on the ward will help to get you ready. A doctor on the ward will explain the procedure to you so that you can sign a consent form. Please ask any questions you wish.

What happens?

You will be asked to lie on your side on the X-ray table. A tube is passed into the rectum and through into the colon until it has crossed the narrowing or blockage. A metallic stent is then put in place to stop the narrowing returning. This will be introduced over a guidewire, and will automatically expand to open up the bowel.

Is it painful?

The procedure can be uncomfortable and therefore sedation and painkillers are given if required.

How long does it take?

The procedure will usually be completed within an hour.

Afterwards

When the procedure is finished you must stay in bed for a couple of hours or until the sedation wears off. You may find you will need to open your bowels on repeated occasions. A nurse will take regular checks of your pulse and blood pressure. If you experience any pain after the dilatation, tell the nurse looking after you, who will give you some painkillers. Laxatives are advised in the diet following the procedure to maintain patency of the stent.

Results

A doctor on the ward will talk to you about the procedure shortly after it.

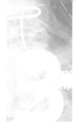

HEPATOBILIARY INTERVENTION

Over the years, hepatobiliary work has evolved into a specialty that requires a multidisciplinary approach, utilizing the skills of the clinician, endoscopist and interventional radiologist. Such collaboration has resulted in improved diagnosis and clinical outcome in this difficult group of patients.

3.1 Bile Duct Obstruction

Presentation

Jaundice

± Pain

± Fever, rigors

Jaundice can be subdivided into congenital, haemolytic hyperbilirubinaemias and cholestatic jaundice. Haemolytic and congenital hyperbilirubinaemias are not a cause of bile duct obstruction.

Cholestatic jaundice can be divided into intrahepatic and extrahepatic cholestasis. Intrahepatic cholestasis is due to underlying parenchymal liver damage or to excretory dysfunction of the bile canaliculi at a cellular level. Extrahepatic cholestasis is due to large duct obstruction resulting in cessation of bile flow at any point in the biliary tract distal to the bile canaliculi.

Common-duct stones		Biliary stricture
Carcinoma:	head of pancreas	Pancreatitis
	ampulla	Sclerosing cholangitis
	bile duct	Nodal compression

Table 3.11 Causes of extrahepatic cholestasis

Investigations

To determine the cause of any underlying jaundice

Full blood count

Clotting screen

Liver function tests

Hepatitis virology screen

Ultrasound – to measure the size of the bile ducts and to visualize the level of the obstruction

Magnetic resonance cholangio-pancreatography (MRCP). This does not involve the injection of a contrast agent but is generated by the high paramagnetic signal produced from the bile (Figure 3.11)

Figure 3.11
There is mild dilatation of the common bile duct (arrow) down to the level of the ampulla, due to an underlying small ampullary tumour

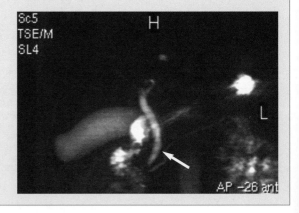

Treatment options

Depends upon the level of the obstruction and the local expertise available

Endoscopic retrograde cholangiography (ERC)

Allows both diagnostic and therapeutic management

Can be technically difficult and is dependent upon conventional anatomy

Tends to be first approach for low bile duct obstruction

Interventional therapy	Percutaneous transhepatic cholangiography (PTC) is still widely used for failed ERCP in low bile duct strictures and in primary management of hilar obstruction
Indications	Failed ERC High lesions
Contraindications	Abnormal blood coagulation profile (INR >1.5; platelets <80 000) requires correction before the procedure can be undertaken
Patient preparation	Informed consent Intravenous access Local anaesthetic + sedation + intravenous analgesia Prophylactic antibiotics
Procedure	Under fluoroscopic guidance, a right-sided/left-sided approach can be performed (ultrasound is of use with both approaches) (Figure 3.12)

Figure 3.12
PTC performed using right-sided approach. There is a common hepatic duct stricture with a blocked endoscopic plastic stent (arrow)

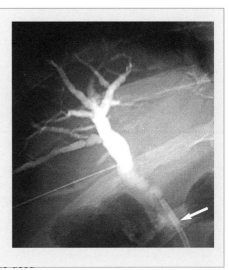

A single capsular puncture is performed in order to reduce the risks of complications

Multiple passes within the liver parenchyma do not appear to be directly correlated with subsequent complications

Right or left sided punctures can be performed. MRCP assists in planning the approach

Non-dilated systems are sometimes punctured for diagnostic purposes. These, though technically more difficult, are still achievable

Entry into the biliary tree is recognized by the slow streaming of contrast

USS guidance assists in puncture of the biliary tree with the minimal number of passes

Having gained entry, a sample of bile is removed and sent for cytological and bacteriological analysis

A cholangiogram is then performed

Stricture management

Having identified an area of narrowing on the cholangiogram, a standard hydrophilic wire is used to negotiate the stenosis (Figure 3.13)

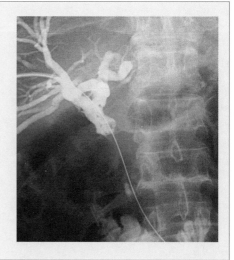

Figure 3.13
Stricture traversed using a guidewire. The Endoscopic stent has been displaced into the duodenum

External/internal biliary drainage is performed by insertion of a drainage catheter and this is usually left on external drainage for 2–3 days (Figure 3.14)

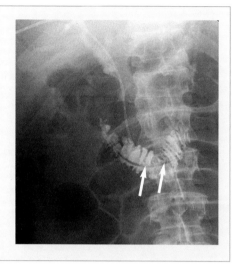

Sometimes, the stenosis is not negotiable in the first instance; however, following 2 days of external drainage, almost all stenoses can be crossed

Formal management of the stricture depending on its nature is discussed in section 3.4

Outcome

Dilated: 100% technical success
Non-dilated: 85% technical success

Complications

Pain
Haemobilia
Pneumothorax
Bile effusion
Biliary peritonitis
Bacteraemia/septicaemia

3.2 Gallstones

Presentation

Found in 10–20% of the population of the Western hemisphere
Twice as common in young women (<40 yrs) as in men, although
the difference decreases with increasing age

Most gallstones are asymptomatic
When they pass into the biliary tract, they can give rise to biliary
obstruction, so producing pain and cholestatic jaundice; added
bacterial infection can occur resulting in cholangitis
Rarely, gallstones can perforate through the gallbladder into the
intestine and become impacted at the terminal ileum, resulting in
gallstone ileus (presenting as small-bowel obstruction)

Investigations

Full blood count
Clotting screen
Liver function tests
Plain abdominal X-ray – gallstone seen in 10% of cases
Ultrasound examination
Nuclear medicine scans – HIDA (Hepatic iminodiacetic acid)
scintigraphy
MRCP

Treatment options

Medical management

In the acute setting with no sequelae suggesting pancreatitis,
conservative management involving rehydration and intravenous
antibiotic therapy is the standard practice

Surgery

After the resolution of acute symptoms, an interval
cholecystectomy can be performed – this may be undertaken
either open or laparoscopically
The advent of laparoscopic techniques has led to a change in
practice as regards known common-bile-duct stones – traditionally,
operative cholangiography was relatively common-place; however,

nowadays, if common-bile-duct stones are shown to be present prior to the cholecystectomy, an ERC with a sphincterotomy is normally undertaken

This has a 95% success rate

There is a 1% risk of bleeding and a 2–4% risk of pancreatitis

Interventional therapy

Percutaneous stone removal is reserved for:

- patients with unconventional anatomy or those who have undergone upper gastrointestinal surgery, so precluding ERC
- patients not suitable for surgical removal with:
    gallbladder stones
    common bile duct stones and failed ERC
- large stones
- strictures and failed ERC
- hepatic stones that are difficult to remove via an endoscopic route

Patient preparation

Informed consent

Intravenous access

Antibiotic prophylaxis

Procedure

A standard PTC is performed

The stones are located

Stone removal is achieved by one of the following:

- mechanical fragmentation
- balloon extrusion
- chemical solution (only applies to cholesterol stones)

If post-operatively a T-tube has been left in situ, to allow a mature tract to form, percutaneous removal should be performed at approximately 4–6 weeks

Rendezvous procedure for stone removal

Undertaken in cases of difficult anatomy (periampullary diverticulum or post-surgical Bilroth type II) or failed ERC

Has the advantage that it negates the need for the formation of a 10–12 F track through the liver

Involves a PTC, which allows the introduction of a guidewire into the biliary system and the placement of its distal end within the duodenum – this enables the endoscopist accurately to identify the position of the ampulla, snare the wire and allow subsequent endoscopic stone removal (Figures 3.21–3.23)

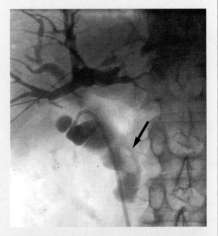

Figure 3.21
Endoscopic drain within the common duct, but system not decompressed. Right sided PTC shows duct dilatation and a hilar stricture (arrow) with filling defect consistent with stone

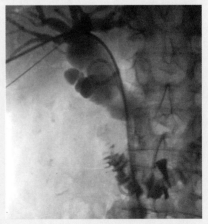

Figure 3.22
Stricture traversed by standard catheter-guidewire technique Endoscopic stent in situ previously placed at rendezvous and no longer accessible due to Roux loop – this had become blocked

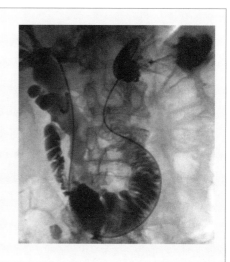

3.3 Gallbladder Problems

Investigations

Full blood count
Clotting screen
Liver function tests
Ultrasound to confirm the presence of gallbladder dilatation with
evidence of acute inflammation (± internal echoes within the
gallbladder suggestive of empyema)

Treatment options

Most gallbladder pathology is treated surgically
Increasingly this is undertaken by laparoscopic cholecystectomy,
although difficult cases (up to 30%) still require open surgery

Interventional therapy

Has a limited role in gallbladder disease per se, but is important
for those patients unfit for surgery. There are two basic techniques:
• fine-needle aspiration of the gallbladder
• percutaneous cholecystotomy

Indications

Fine-needle aspiration
of the gallbladder

To allow cytological analysis and culture of the bile, so enabling accurate diagnosis and appropriate antimicrobial therapy

Percutaneous
cholecystotomy

Decompression and drainage of acute cholecystitis/empyema in surgically unfit patients

Alternative route for biliary drainage

Access tract for stone extraction or dissolution

Can be useful in ITU (intensive therapy unit) patients with unknown sepsis – 60% show improvement following cholecystostomy secondary to acalculous cholecystitis

Patient preparation

Informed consent

Intravenous access ± sedation and local anaesthetic

Prophylactic antibiotics

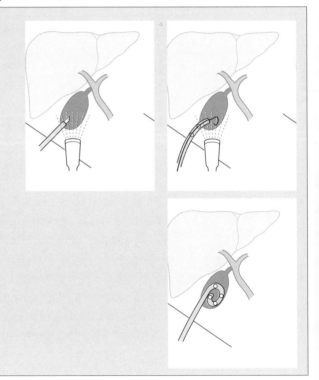

Figure 3.31
The gall bladder is punctured under ultrasound guidance (Seldinger technique)

Figure 3.32
The pigtail catheter is introduced over the guidewire, following dilatation of the tract

Figure 3.33
The guidewire is withdrawn leaving the self-retaining pigtail catheter inserted in the gall bladder

Procedure	Aseptic technique under ultrasound guidance
	Transperitoneal or transhepatic route is used
	Sample of bile is removed and sent for cytological analysis and culture
	A locking pigtail catheter is placed within the gallbladder and left on open drainage (Figures 3.31–3.33)
Outcome	Outcome depends on patient's condition at presentation
	Interval formal cholecystectomy can be performed when the patient's general health has improved
Complications	Biliary peritonitis
	Pain
	Bacteraemia/septicaemia

3.4 Biliary Strictures

Presentation

Jaundice ± pain

Pale stools, dark urine

± Fever, rigors

Benign strictures	Malignant strictures
Iatrogenic (post-surgical, 95%)	Carcinoma of the pancreas
Chronic pancreatitis	Bile-duct tumours
Sclerosing cholangitis	Extrahepatic nodal disease
Biliary calculi	

Table 3.41 Causes of benign and malignant strictures

Investigations

Blood tests (full blood count, clotting screen, renal and liver function tests)

Ultrasound

MRCP

CT

Endoscopy

Treatment options

Endoscopy	Can be both diagnostic and therapeutic (sphincterotomy, stents)

Surgical	Resection (Whipple's)
	Bypass

Interventional therapy Normally reserved for those patients who are unsuitable for surgical management
Endoscopic access is the procedure of choice for low bile duct strictures, with PTC reserved for endoscopic failures. PTC should be the procedure of choice for hilar strictures

Patient preparation	Informed consent
	Intravenous access
	Sedation + local anaesthetic
	Antibiotic prophylaxis

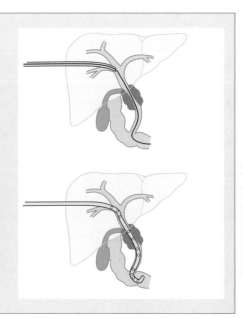

Figure 3.41
Following right-sided approach, a biliary manipulation catheter and guidewire are used to negotiate the lumen of the stricture

Figure 3.42
Internal/external biliary drainage with proximal side hole above the stricture

Procedure	Initially, a PTC is performed and biliary drainage achieved
	If the diagnosis of inoperable malignancy is made, primary metallic stenting can be undertaken. If diagnosis is not known, external drainage can be carried out for 2–3 days
	Bile is sent for cytological analysis and culture, to confirm the diagnosis and assist with antimicrobial therapy (Figure 3.41, 3.42) Subsequent plastic stent (benign) or metallic stent (malignant) insertion can be undertaken
Benign strictures	Traditionally treated by balloon angioplasty or surgery (either primarily or following primary or secondary failure of balloon dilatation) Balloon angioplasty allows repeated treatments If resistant, a 4 F catheter can be left across the stricture for 1 month, so allowing access if the stricture reforms
Outcome	80% success at 30 months 55% success at 5 years
Complications	Bacteraemia/septicaemia Biliary leak

Figure 3.43
PTC performed using right-sided approach, following a period of external drainage. Common hepatic duct stricture seen with blocked endoscopic stent

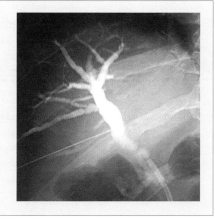

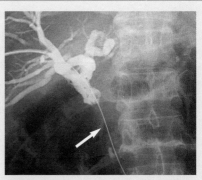

Figure 3.44
Stricture traversed using a guidewire (arrow). Following balloon dilatation, primary stent placement can be performed. If the diagnosis is unknown internal/external drainage can be instituted

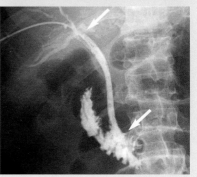

Figure 3.45
Mesh metal expandable biliary stent from the level of the duct confluence to the ampulla (arrow). System decompressed and freely draining

Malignant strictures

Formal treatment is only undertaken once cytological diagnosis has been confirmed

Strictures are traversed with the standard guidewire/catheter technique. If the diagnosis needs to be confirmed a period of external/internal drainage can be instituted (Figures 3.43–3.45)

Plastic and metal biliary stents are available

Plastic stents	Metal stents
12 F transhepatic tract	7 F transhepatic tract
Increased risk of haemobilia, migration,	Increase patency
patient discomfort at deployment	Expensive
Reduced patency	Non-removable
Two-stage procedure	
Allows exchange	

Table 3.42 Characteristics of plastic and metal stents

Outcome	Long-term stent patency:
	• plastic stents – 126 days
	• metal stents – 273 days

Complications	Patient discomfort/pain at time of deployment
	Haemobilia
	Stent-related complications:
	• plastic stents – migration (3–10%), occlusion (6–25%)
	• metal stents – tumour overgrowth (7–14%)

3.5 Liver Biopsy

In patients with a normal coagulation profile, liver biopsy is a ward-based procedure with low morbidity

The role of image guidance is to:
• increase the yield, especially involving small focal lesions
• further reduce the risks of pneumothorax or damage to adjacent structures

Investigations	Full blood count
	Clotting screen
	Liver function tests
	Ultrasound

| Interventional therapy | Has its main role in the group of patients with an abnormal coagulation screen, in whom there is a significant risk of bleeding post biopsy |

INR	Treatment
1.0–1.4	Correction of factors
1.5–2.0	Plugged biopsy or transjugular
>2.0	Transvenous approach (transjugular)

Table 3.51 Treatment options based on INR values

Patient preparation	Informed consent
	Intravenous access
	Local anaesthetic ± sedation
	Correction of factors: vitamin K
	FFP (fresh frozen plasma)

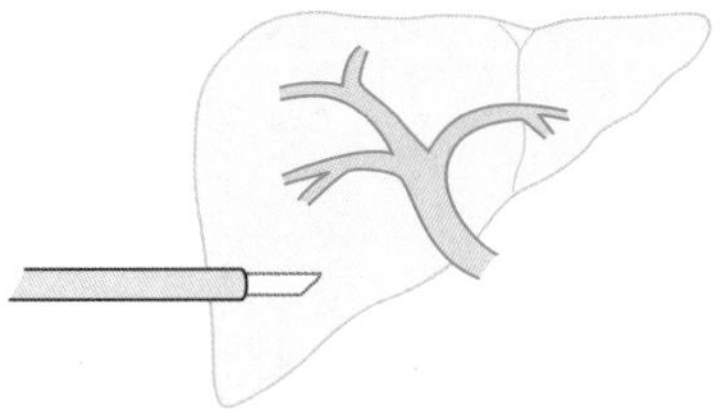

Figure 3.51
Core biopsy performed
with tru-cut needle
through a sheath

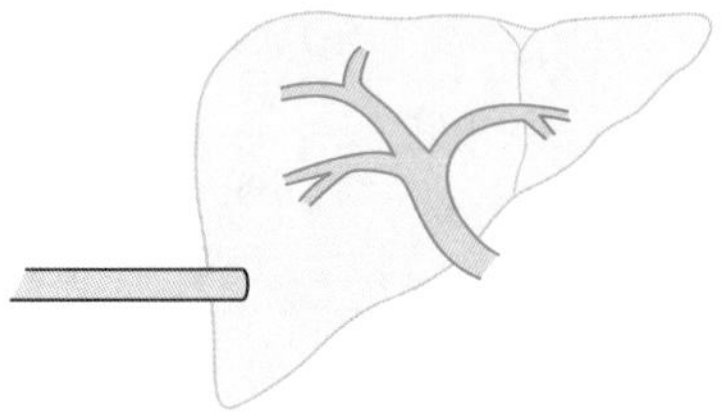

Figure 3.52
Sheaths left in situ

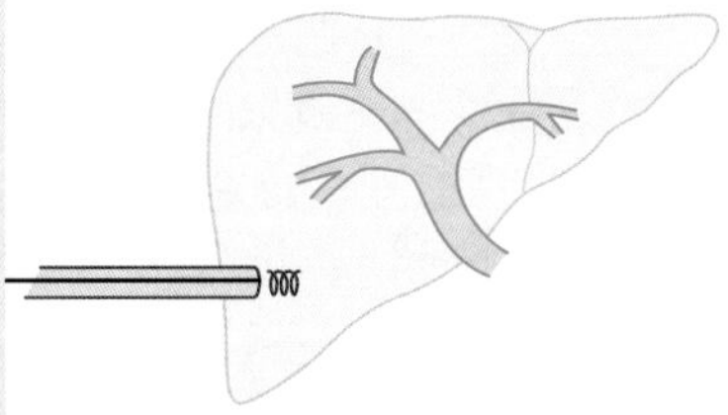

Figure 3.53
The biopsy tract is
embolized with steel coils

Plugged biopsy	The biopsy is performed using a standard needle/sheath
(INR 1.5–2.0)	technique (Figure 3.51, 3.52)
	After the biopsy, the tract is embolized using particulate material –
	steel coils (Figure 3.53)

| Outcome | Minimum morbidity/mortality |
| | Technical success rate 98% |

Complications	Persistent bleeding:

Persistent bleeding:
- necessitates arteriography ± further embolization
- cardiovascular instability
- may require surgical intervention

Transvenous approach
(INR>2.0)

i) Transjugular route

A low internal jugular approach is performed using image guidance (ultrasound) (Figure 3.54)

Access to the liver parenchyma is gained via the hepatic veins, under fluoroscopic control

An 18 G biopsy is performed

A check venogram is performed to ensure there is no extracapsular leak

Outcome

Technical success rate 98% (failure in patients with large volume ascites, small liver)

Complications

Capsular perforation (4.0%); no sequelae
Significant haemorrhage (0.4%)
Infection (0.1%)

Figure 3.54
A vascular sheath and guidewire is introduced via a right internal jugular vein. Hepatic vein venogram demonstrates normal liver anatomy. This allows introduction of a 7 F TJ needle

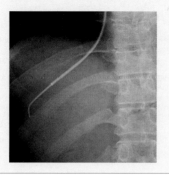
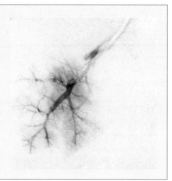

If transjugular route not possible due to bilateral IJV occlusion it is possible to perform a transfemoral approach with biopsy forceps

3.6 Variceal Bleeding

Presentation

Uncontrollable haematemesis secondary to liver disease. This includes high-risk patients with known varices awaiting liver transplantation

Investigations

Full blood screen
Ultrasound
CT

Treatment options

Endoscopy

Banding
Sclerotherapy

Surgical shunts

Splenorenal
Mesocaval

Interventional therapy

Transjugular intrahepatic porto-systemic shunt (TIPS), which was first developed in 1988, has now evolved into a well-established technique for a specific group of patients

Contraindications

Absolute

Right heart failure
Pulmonary/ascitic sepsis
Extensive malignancy involving liver vessels/parenchyma

Relative

Portal vein occlusion (Budd-Chiari syndrome)

Patient preparation

Informed consent
Intravenous access
Local anaesthetic + sedation
Antibiotic cover

Procedure

Under aseptic technique and fluoroscopic control, a transjugular approach to the right and middle hepatic veins is performed

A tract is created between the hepatic vein and the intrahepatic portion of the right portal vein (this is aided by CO_2 portography, splenoportography or ultrasound) (Figure 3.61)

The tract is dilated by ballooning (Figure 3.62)

An expandable metallic stent is used to form the portosystemic shunt (Figure 3.63)

The gradient should be reduced by approximately 10–15 mmHg

Figure 3.61
Needle and guidewire advanced using various imaging techniques from the hepatic vein into the portal vein

Figure 3.62
Balloon angioplasty is used to dilate a liver tract connecting the two venous systems

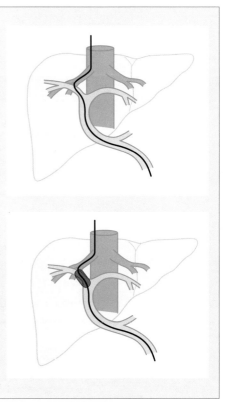

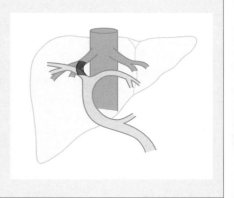

Figure 3.63
Expandable metal stent is
deployed along the liver
tract

Outcome

Technical success rate 95–100% with a procedural time of
approximately 1–2 h
Shunt malfunction occurs in 25–40% at 1–6 months (due to
underlying intimal hyperplasia)
Re-intervention rate at 6 months is 25%; at 1 year, 50%; at
2 years, 65%
Secondary stent patency rate is approximately 100% (involves the
use of Doppler ultrasound surveillance)

Complications

Mortality (1–10%)
Peritoneal haemorrhage (1–6%)
Haemobilia (1–14%)
Sepsis (10%)
Hepatic encephalopathy – especially if the gradient is less than
10 mmHg (25%)

PERCUTANEOUS CHOLANGIOGRAPHY AND DRAINAGE

What is percutaneous cholangiography and drainage

This is a test performed in the X-ray department that allows us to look at the drainage of bile from the liver. At the same time the bile ducts can be drained if necessary.

Preparation

In the X-ray department you will be expected to lie flat on your back on an X-ray table.

What happens?

Under local anaesthetic and X-ray control, a fine needle will be introduced into the liver, through the right side of your abdomen. Once the bile ducts are seen, a tube is normally left in place to drain the liver. The tube is stitched in place and attached to a drainage bag fixed to your gown.

If a narrowing is seen, it can be stretched by a balloon and may be kept open by a plastic tube or stent ('spring').

How long will it take?

The procedure will usually take 30–90 min.

Is it painful?

You will be given oxygen and can have a sedative injection via a vein in your hand. This will make you sleepy, but will still allow you to co-operate during the procedure.

Afterwards

You will not be able to start eating or drinking for 6 h post procedure. During this time you will be kept on a drip and under regular nursing observations.

Results

At 2–3 days, you may return to the X-ray department for a check X-ray and, if necessary, further treatment.

TRANSJUGULAR/TRANSFEMORAL BIOPSY

What is a transjugular/ transfemoral biopsy

Liver samples are usually taken through the skin (percutaneously) unless the blood is not clotting properly. If this is the case, a safe way of obtaining the sample is by a transjugular (TJ) (or rarely transfemoral) route.

Preparation

The nurses on the ward will help you to get ready. You must not eat for 2 h before the examination. A doctor from the ward will explain the procedure to you so that you can sign a consent form before you come down to the X-ray department. Please ask any questions you wish.

What happens?

This involves a small tube (catheter) being introduced, under local anaesthetic, into a vein in the neck, if a transjugular route is to be used, or via a vein in the groin, if a transfemoral route is desirable. The catheter is then moved into the liver. The X-ray machine is used to show that the catheter is in the correct place to take the biopsy and this will move around you during the procedure.

How long will it take?

The procedure will be completed usually within an hour and you will have to lie flat on your back during this time.

Is it painful?

An injection of local anaesthetic is given into the skin of the neck or groin, which will sting initially but will quickly make the area go numb. You will then only be aware of a pushing sensation as the catheter is moved in and out.

Afterwards

When the test is finished the tube will be removed and the doctor will press on this area of the neck or groin until the bleeding stops. You will probably get a bruise in this area. You will have to stay in bed for about 6 h and a nurse will take regular checks of your pulse and blood pressure.

Results

The samples that are taken have to be sent to histology and the doctor on the ward will be able to tell you the results when he/she receives them in a couple of days.

TIPS (TRANSJUGULAR INTRAHEPATIC PORTO-SYSTEMIC SHUNT)

What is TIPS?

This is an X-ray procedure to improve the flow of blood within the liver, by connecting different blood supplies.

Preparation

The nurses on the ward will help you to get ready. You should not have anything to eat or drink for 4 h before the examination. A doctor on the ward will explain the procedure to you and you will need to sign a consent form. Please ask any questions you wish.

What happens?

A doctor will feed a small tube (catheter) into a blood vessel within the neck. This is then moved into the liver, and a metal spring (stent) is released and left inside the liver to relieve blood pressures within the liver itself. The X-ray machine is used to show the blood vessels and catheter, as it is moved into position, and the machine will move around you into various positions to take the pictures. In the X-ray department you will be expected to lie flat on your back on an X-ray table.

How long will it take?

The procedure is usually completed within 2–3 h, although occasionally it may take a little longer.

Is it painful?

You will be given oxygen and can have a sedative injection via a vein in your hand. This will make you sleepy, but will still allow you to co-operate during the procedure.

Before the tube is inserted into the vessel within the neck, an injection of local anaesthetic is given into the skin. This will sting at first but will soon go numb and you should then only be aware of a pushing sensation. Some contrast (X-ray dye) will also be introduced at various intervals, which may give you a warm feeling. This is completely normal.

Afterwards

When the test is finished, the catheter will be removed and the doctor will press on this area of the neck until the bleeding stops. You will probably get a bruise in this area. When you are back in your bed, a nurse will take regular checks of your pulse and blood pressure and this will continue on the ward. You will need to lie flat in bed for a few hours.

Results

A doctor on your ward will talk to you about the procedure shortly after it.

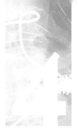

URORADIOLOGICAL INTERVENTION

All parts of the urinary tract are accessible by percutaneous routes
The translumbar approach is best for the kidneys and ureters,
whilst a lower abdominal approach is best for the bladder
All modalities can be used to provide guidance, the most
frequently used being ultrasound
There is minimum morbidity, and technical success rates are high

4.1 Renal Cysts

Presentation

Common asymptomatic finding
Large cysts can present as symptomatic swellings that cause both
discomfort and, occasionally, pain
As a result of high-quality ultrasound and CT, most cystic lesions
within the kidneys can be positively diagnosed as simple cysts,
thus requiring no further investigation

Exceptions to this are:
- if the question of malignant change is raised
- if the diagnostic criteria necessary for the diagnosis of a simple
  cyst cannot be confirmed

Investigations

Ultrasound
Contrast-enhanced CT
Spiral CT with a reduced field of view

Treatment options

The procedure of open cyst biopsy and aspiration is not always
necessary as percutaneous techniques have high success rates and
are associated with minimum morbidity

Interventional therapy	Renal cyst aspiration ± ablation
Contraindications	Bleeding diatheses
Patient preparation	Informed consent – stating risk of pneumothorax and damage to neighbouring organs
	Local anaesthesia ± sedation
Procedure	Aseptic technique
	Patient is placed prone
	Under ultrasound/CT/fluoroscopic guidance, an 18–22 G needle is used to perform aspiration
	Fluid is sent for analysis
	If ablation is required, this is normally done at a second sitting, once cytological analysis has confirmed the diagnosis
	Ablation is achieved by local injection of alcohol, following percutaneous aspiration (Figures 4.11–4.14)
Outcome	Technical success rate approximately 98%

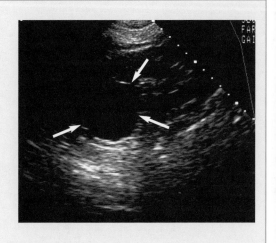

Figure 4.11
Ultrasound showing a large renal cyst of the upper pole of the right kidney

Complications	Haematoma formation
	Retroperitoneal haemorrhage
	Pneumothorax

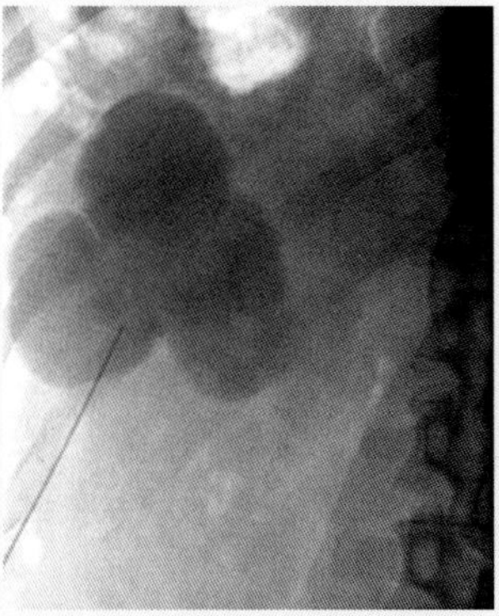

Figure 4.12
The cyst has been
punctured percutaneously

Figure 4.13
A drainage catheter has
been introduced to allow
drainage and alcohol
administration

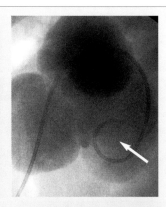

Figure 4.14
Post ablation of cyst

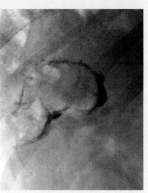

4.2 Urinary Obstruction

Presentation

Flank pain radiating to the groin
Associated haematuria ± fever, leucocytosis or pyuria
Deteriorating renal function
Demonstrable hydronephrosis

Causes are multiple and include:

- calculi
- mass/tumour
- retroperitoneal fibrosis
- bladder outflow obstruction
- neurological deficit

Investigations

Ultrasound

Intravenous urogram (IVU)

Nuclear medicine scans – MAG3 or DMSA

Treatment options

- Surgical nephrostomy
- Retrograde double J stent insertion, following cystoscopy
- Percutaneous drainage
- Antegrade percutaneous double J stent insertion

The type of treatment undertaken is dependent on local services, patient suitability and the underlying pathology

Interventional therapy

Percutaneous nephrostomy

Percutaneous antegrade pigtail double J stent insertion

Contraindications

Absolute

None

Relative

Bleeding diatheses

Inability to lie prone

Patient preparation

Informed consent

Local anaesthetic ± sedation

Appropriate antibiotic cover

Procedure   A 22 G needle is introduced under ultrasound control into the collecting systems and antegrade pyelography performed – this allows percutaneous access

The obstructed systems are decompressed to reduce the risk of subsequent urosepsis

The systems are then opacified and percutaneous drainage achieved through a mid or lower pole posterior calyx using a pigtail catheter

A Seldinger technique (see appendix) is used for the placement of all nephrostomy catheters (Figures 4.21–4.25)

Figure 4.21
Opacified collecting
system with stone in
proximal ureter (arrow)

Figure 4.22
Pigtail catheter in situ
within the right renal
pelvis

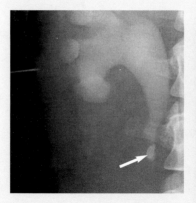
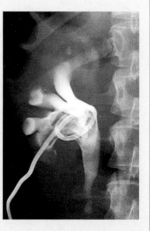

Figure 4.23
Under ultrasound control, a 22 G needle is introduced into the collecting systems, which are then opacified

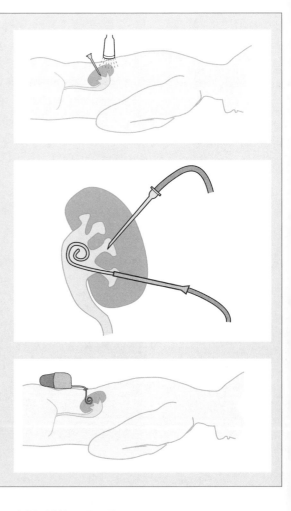

Figure 4.24
Using a Seldinger technique (see appendix), a pigtail catheter is inserted through a lower pole calyx

Figure 4.25
The dilated system is drained and the external drainage bag attached to the patient's clothing

Outcome

Success rate of 95–98% in the dilated system
Only 3–5% of percutaneous nephrostomies require prolonged hospitalization, compared with 25% of surgical nephrostomies

Complications

Pneumothorax, urinoma or haemorrhage (1–2%)
Urosepsis (7% risk of septic shock)

4.3 Renal Calculi

Presentation

Asymptomatic – incidental finding

Symptomatic – present with features of urinary obstruction, infection, renal damage

Investigations

Ultrasound

IVU

Nuclear medicine scans

CT

Treatment options

Conservative management 5-mm stones usually pass spontaneously

Extracorporeal lithotripsy 85–90% successful but usually requires several treatment courses

Other treatment options are still necessary, especially if the stones are:

- composed of cystine or calcium phosphate
- situated proximal to an obstruction of the urinary tract (diverticulum – stenosis)
- greater than 2.5 cm in diameter within a normal collecting system

Interventional therapy

Percutaneous nephrolithotomy is the primary treatment for staghorn calculi and stones resistant to lithotripsy. It is usually performed as a combined procedure in the operating theatre with the urologist

The interventional radiologist will usually create a 30–32 F access tract to the calculus with the subsequent endoscopic removal of the stone being performed by the urologist

The same technique of nephrolithotomy can be used to undertake renal biopsy, tumour or foreign body removal, as well as the treatment of PUJ (pelvico-ureteric junction) obstruction and infundibular stenoses

| Patient preparation | Informed consent |
| | General anaesthesia or epidural anaesthesia is required to provide sufficient pain control |

Procedure	Can be performed in one or two stages
	If over two stages, there is normally a delay of several days to allow maturation of the tract formed at the initial dilatation
	The two-stage procedure is associated with less haemorrhage and therefore easier endoscopic intervention

One-stage procedure	An antegrade pyelogram is performed to provide a calyceal map (Figure 4.31)
	A tract is established and dilated over a guidewire to 30–32 F (10 mm) using dilators or high-pressure balloons (Figure 4.32)
	Multiple tracts may be necessary if a staghorn calculus is being treated
	Endoscopic intervention is undertaken, with calculi being fragmented by ultrasonics, laser lithotripsy or electrohydraulics
	The fragments are then removed by a Dormier basket
	Any residual fragments can be dispersed using extracorporeal lithotripsy (Figure 4.33, 4.34)

| Outcome | Technical success rate 90–95% |
| | This increases further with follow-up lithotripsy |

Figure 4.31
An antegrade pyelogram is performed showing a large calculus within the renal pelvis (arrow). The lower pole calyx has been punctured percutaneously

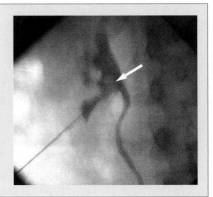

Complications   Renal haemorrhage (12%)

Arteriovenous fistula/pseudoaneurysm (1%)

Urosepsis (1–2%)

Pneumothorax (0.1%)

Damage to adjacent organs or bowel (0.01%)

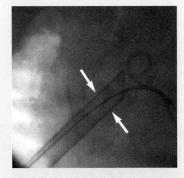

Figure 4.32
A tract is formed and dilated to 30–32 F (10 mm)

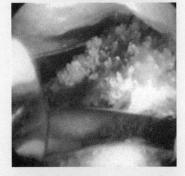

Figure 4.33
The stone is removed by surgical forceps having been crushed

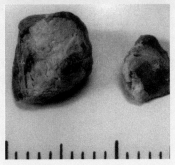

Figure 4.34
The stone fragments

4.4 Urinary Strictures

Presentation
Urinary obstruction
Haematuria
Deteriorating renal function

Investigations
Ultrasound
IVU
Nuclear medicine scans
CT
MRI (magnetic resonance imaging)

Treatment options
Urinary tract obstruction is preferably approached from below,
as a general principle
Retrograde cystoscopic balloon dilatation and double J stent insertion
Antegrade nephrostomy, balloon dilatation and double
J stent insertion

Benign strictures
If newly formed (less than 3 months), can be successfully treated
with balloon dilatation
Strictures secondary to surgery, radiotherapy, vascularized
segments, as well as ureteric strictures or strictures involving a
transplanted kidney, have a low success with balloon dilatation,
and ureteric stenting should be considered

Malignant strictures
Require primary stenting

Interventional therapy
Reserved for cases in which cystoscopic treatment has failed

Contraindications
Bleeding diatheses

Patient preparation
Informed consent
Local anaesthesia ± sedation

Procedure
An antegrade pyelogram is performed to provide a calyceal map

A percutaneous nephrostomy tract is formed via a mid or upper pole calyx

This allows a good direction of access to the ureters to allow balloon dilatation or stenting

1. Balloon dilatation

It is essential to exclude the possibility of the stricture being malignant prior to treatment, by brush biopsies and radiological evaluation with CT or MRI

Procedure

Balloon dilatation to approximately 4–6 mm is undertaken. An 8–10 F urethral stent is left in situ for approximately 2 weeks – this allows healing of the stricture and reduces the risk of recurrence (Figure 4.41–4.43)

At 2 weeks, the stent is removed and a nephrostomy catheter placed within the renal pelvis – this allows continued drainage of the system while the oedema surrounding the ureteric narrowing resolves

This procedure can be repeated on multiple occasions

Outcome

Technical success rate in excess of 95%

Long-term results are variable

Figure 4.41
An antegrade nephrostogram showing a right distal ureteric stricture (arrow)

Figure 4.42
Balloon dilatation of the ureteric stricture (arrow)

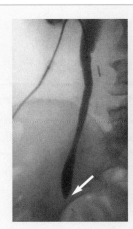
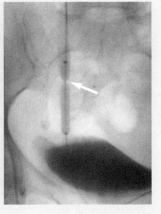

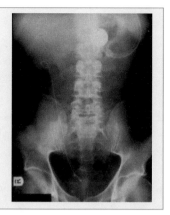

Figure 4.43
A double J stent is left in situ for several weeks to maintain ureteral patency

Complications	Urethral perforation or intimal disruption can occur rarely – if this arises, stenting is performed
2. Ureteric stenting	Normally undertaken for malignant strictures, ureteric perforation or specific longstanding benign strictures that have proved resistant to balloon dilatation
Procedure	The access technique is the same as that for balloon dilatation Following this, a JJ ureteric stent is placed The distal pigtail is formed within the bladder, the proximal pigtail within the renal pelvis A percutaneous nephrostomy is left in situ, but can usually be removed at 24 h
Outcome	Patency rate at 3 months is 95%; at 6 months, 54% Ureteric stents require periodic re-evaluation using renal sonography and renal function tests – replacement is advised every 3–4 months. Once an antegrade stent has been positioned, replacement stents can usually be introduced via a retrograde route (cystoscopy) New metallic stents for use in the genitourinary system have recently been introduced – their long-term evaluation is awaited

Complications	As for balloon dilatation
	Malposition/migration of the stents
	Inability to cross a tight malignant stricture

4.5 Urinary Retention

Presentation	Inability to pass urine
	Abdominal discomfort
	Can be asymptomatic if chronic in nature
	Secondary to prostate enlargement, urethral strictures, pelvic trauma and neuropathic bladder
Investigations	Ultrasound
	Renal function tests
Treatment options	Surgical cystotomy is only undertaken as part of formal surgical intervention
Interventional therapy	Percutaneous suprapubic cystostomy is the treatment of choice
Contraindications	
Absolute	None
Relative	Bleeding diathesis
Patient preparation	Informed consent
	Local anaesthetic
Procedure	The patient is placed supine
	Under aseptic technique, a suprapubic approach via a paramedian line of insertion is performed
	Ultrasound is used to assess the size of the bladder and the presence of small-bowel loops within the pelvis

A 20 G needle puncture is introduced, the tract is dilated to 20 F, and a Foley balloon catheter is placed within the bladder

If long-term catheterization is required, a catheter of at least 16 F dimension should be used (Figures 4.51–4.54)

Outcome

Technical success rate 100%

Complications

Transient haematuria

Urinary tract infection

Small risk to adjacent loops of small bowel

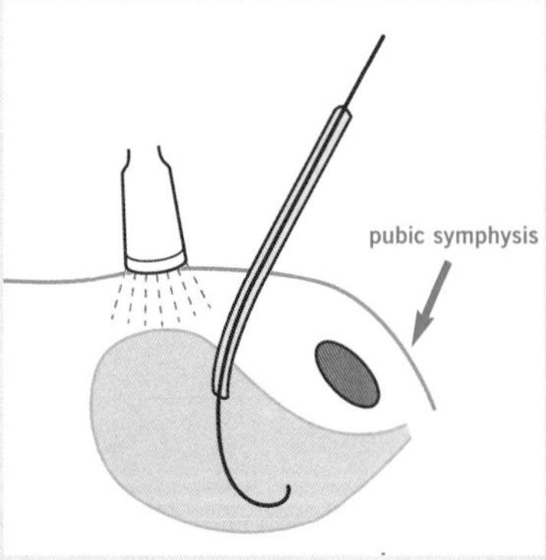

Figure 4.51
Under ultrasound guidance the bladder is visualized and a guidewire advanced into the lumen

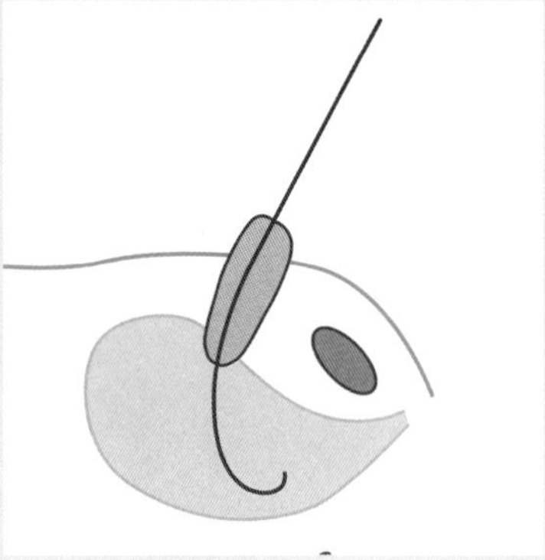

pubic symphysis

Figure 4.52
The tract is balloon dilated

Figure 4.53
A peel-away sheath is in
place and a Foley catheter
has been advanced into
the bladder

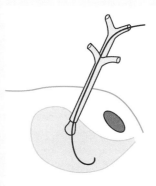

Figure 4.54
Foley catheter in place
with balloon inflated

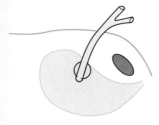

NEPHROSTOMY/NEPHROSTOGRAM

What is a nephrostomy/ nephrostogram?

This is an examination, using ultrasound and X-rays, which gives the doctors detailed information about your kidneys. As your kidneys cannot be shown on X-rays alone, a special X-ray dye known as 'contrast' is also used to create a full and detailed picture. This will be introduced via a needle in the back.

Preparation

The nurses on the ward will help you to get ready. You must not eat for 2 h before the examination, and a doctor on the ward will explain the procedure to you so that you can sign a consent form. You will also be given some antibiotics to prevent infection during the examination.

Is it painful?

You will be given oxygen and can have a sedative and painkilling injection via a vein in your hand. This will make you sleepy, but will still allow you to co-operate during the procedure.

What happens?

In the X-ray department you will be expected to lie on your front on an X-ray table. An injection of local anaesthetic is given into the skin of the abdomen, on the problem side. A needle is then introduced through the skin and into the kidney. The X-ray dye is then injected and some pictures are taken to show how well the kidney is draining. If the kidney is blocked, a small tube is placed over the needle and left within the kidney. The other end outside the abdomen is attached to a small bag, which collects the urine. This system allows the kidney to drain properly. This is called a nephrostomy.

You will be required to come back to the X-ray department in a couple of days so that more X-ray contrast can be injected into the tube to see whether the kidney is improving. This is called a nephrostogram.

How long will it take? The initial procedure will usually be completed within an hour and this also applies to subsequent visits. Initially you may also have an ultrasound scan so that the doctor can accurately locate the kidneys. You will be expected to lie flat on your stomach for the duration of the procedures.

Afterwards You will be required to stay in bed for 12 h after the initial procedure and a nurse will take regular checks of your pulse and blood pressure.

Results The doctor doing the procedure will tell you what they are doing and are going to do. A full discussion with your ward doctor will ensure you understand the results of the test.

VASCULAR INTERVENTION

Venous Intervention

5.1 Access/Lines

The ability of the interventional radiologist to gain venous access in a variety of clinical settings has led to the 'venous access' service becoming an ever-increasing part of the daily workload. This role, originally allocated to surgeons, has been increasingly performed by radiologists for the following reasons:

- Central venous puncture is safer under image guidance
- Radiologists are well practised with wire and catheter techniques
- There is usually a better standard of fluoroscopy in radiology departments than in main operating theatres, so allowing better imaging

Investigations

Full blood count
Clotting time

Indications

Oncology patients requiring systemic chemotherapy or blood products
Haematological patients undergoing bone marrow transplantation
Patients on long-term total parenteral nutrition
Renal patients requiring venous access for dialysis

Types of catheter

Peripherally inserted central venous catheters (Figure 5.11):
- last 2–10 weeks

- useful for outpatient intravenous therapy

Long-term venous access catheters (Figure 5.12):
- types depend upon usage

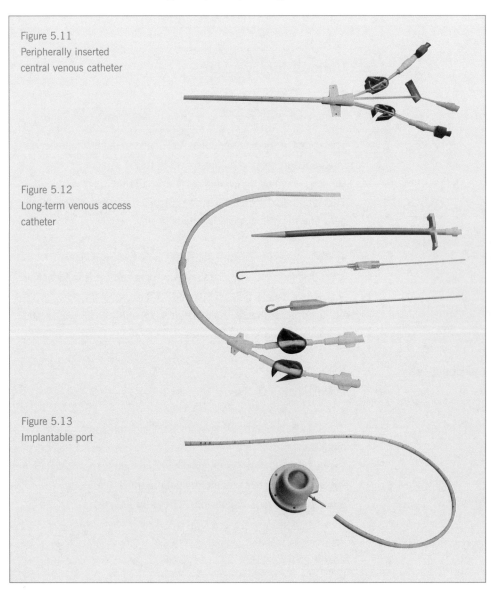

Figure 5.11
Peripherally inserted
central venous catheter

Figure 5.12
Long-term venous access
catheter

Figure 5.13
Implantable port

- single or multiple lumens

Implantable ports (Figure 5.13):
- long-term intravenous blood-product therapy

Patient preparation

Informed consent

Thorough iodine/chlorhexidine scrub, from the level of the mandible to the umbilicus, on the ward

This is then repeated in the interventional suite before commencement of the procedure

Intravenous access for sedation

Correction of abnormal platelet counts/bleeding time

Antibiotic cover

Access via internal jugular vein (IJV)

Procedure

USS guided puncture is used – this is associated with a reduction in catheter-related problems, as well as an increase in both patient comfort and aesthetics (able to hide line position below clothing)

A low approach is performed under image guidance (ultrasound) to offset the increased risks of pneumothorax and an incompressible arterial puncture

Puncture of the IJV is aided by placing the patient 'head down' and by asking the patient to perform a Valsalva manoeuvre

Having gained access, the wire is advanced under fluoroscopic control into the inferior vena cava (IVC)

A percutaneous tunnel of approximately 6 cm is made in an inferolateral direction relative to the puncture site

The central venous line is positioned under fluoroscopic control such that the tip of the line lies at the level of the right atrium

This is then carefully fixed in position and the neck puncture site is sutured

If a port is used, a subcutaneous pocket is made at the level of pectoralis major and is fixed in place with a permanent suture (Figures 5.14–5.16)

Figure 5.14
Needle puncture of the
right IJV under ultrasound
guidance

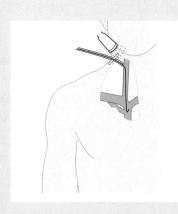

Figure 5.15
The catheter is introduced
under fluoroscopy and
placed such that the tip
lies at the level of the right
atrium

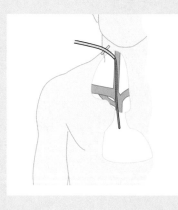

Figure 5.16
A percutaneous tunnel is
formed in an inferolateral
direction and the catheter
exited through a small skin
incision

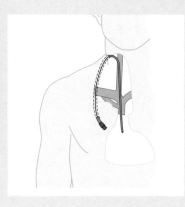

| Outcome | Significant reductions in the risk of low puncture are achieved using real-time ultrasound for needle guidance |
| | There is a high technical success rate, in excess of 98%, providing there is patent venous access |

Complications	Arterial puncture – common carotid/vertebral artery
	Pneumothorax/hydrothorax
	Cervical haematoma/respiratory obstruction
	Nerve palsy – recurrent laryngeal/phrenic
	Tracheal puncture/oesophageal damage

Subclavian venous access

Procedure	A left-sided approach is better because of a straight line of access
	If the right side is used, the sheath needs to be shaped to give a curve of approximately 90°
	A needle puncture is performed using real-time ultrasound, fluoroscopy or following upper limb venography
	Having gained access, the remainder of the procedure is as for IJV puncture (Figures 5.17–5.19)

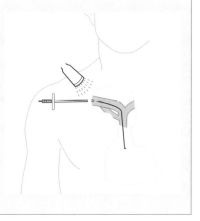

Figure 5.17
Needle puncture is
performed using real-time
ultrasound and the
guidewire inserted

Figure 5.18
The catheter is introduced
under fluoroscopic control

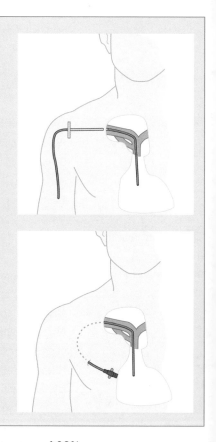

Figure 5.19
A subcutaneous tunnel is
formed and the catheter
exited through the skin

Outcome	Technical success rate is in excess of 98%
Complications	As per IJV puncture, excluding problems associated with the carotid artery
Other routes	External jugular vein Femoral vein Peripheral (via basilic/cephalic veins) IVC – long-term access in patients with occlusion of the superior vena cava (SVC)

Early	Catheter misplacement
	Air embolism
Late	Infection
	Fibrin-sheath formation (can be treated by low-dose thrombolysis/stripping)
	Catheter failure

Table 5.11 Line-associated complications

5.2 Deep-Vein Thrombosis (DVT)/ Pulmonary Embolism (PE)

Presentation

DVT

Classically presents with calf swelling associated with tenderness and pain

History of immobilization, recent surgery or malignancy

Up to 25% of cases occur in symptomless lower limbs

PE

Classically presents with chest pain, hypoxia and haemoptysis

Can be asymptomatic

Approximately 30% of patients have normal chest X-rays and no ECG changes

Investigations

Full blood screen including coagulopathies

D-dimer test – highly sensitive (95%) non-specific test for the presence of venous thrombus

Doppler ultrasound

V/Q scan

CT pulmonary angiogram (Λ dynamic spiral CT examination with high degree of sensitivity to 4th order vessels) A recent development, and gaining in use (Figure 5.21, 5.22)

Treatment options

Medical management is the mainstay of treatment

Comprises immediate anticoagulation with intravenous heparin followed by formal anticoagulation with warfarin

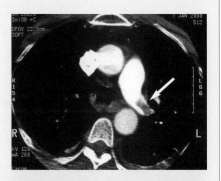

Figure 5.21
Contrast enhanced CT
showing pulmonary
thrombus within the
left pulmonary trunk
(arrow)

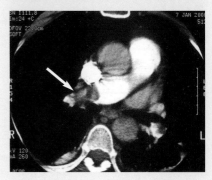

Figure 5.22
Extensive thrombus
within the right
pulmonary trunk
(arrow)

Interventional therapy   IVC filters have an increasing role in individuals with DVT and PE
This group have absolute and relative indications

Indications
Absolute

Patients with PE in spite of adequate anticoagulation
Patients with iliofemoral DVT in whom anticoagulation
is contraindicated
Patients in whom anticoagulation has been ceased because
of complications

Relative
(prophylactic indications)

High-risk patients
Patients requiring surgery who have a known DVT or previous DVT
with PE
Trauma patients with potential long periods of immobilization

Pregnant women with known DVT undergoing labour or possible caesarean section

Types of IVC filters	Permanent
	Permanent retrievable
	Temporary
Patient preparation	Informed consent
	Local anaesthetic
	IVC access

Figure 5.23
IVC venogram via the right common femoral vein.
There is a thrombus occluding the left common iliac vein (arrow).
The position of the renal veins is noted (▶) as the filter is whenever possible placed below the renal veins

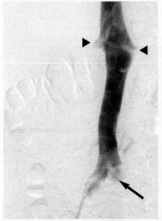
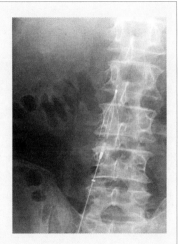

Figure 5.24
Release of the Gunther tulip filter

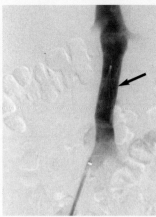

Figure 5.25
Check venogram showing good filter position within the infra-renal IVC

Procedure	Right internal jugular or femoral vein approach
	A contrast venogram is performed to show the level of the renal veins and the extent of the thrombus
	The filter is deployed below the level of the renal veins (exceptions – pregnancy, thrombus within or beyond the renal veins)
	(Figures 5.23–5.25)

| Outcome | There has been no randomized controlled study looking at the efficacy of IVC filters |

Complications	Venous thrombosis at the access site
	Filter migration
	Caval thrombosis (symptomatic in 3–9%)
	Recurrent PE (0.5–7.0%)
	Filter fracture/stent perforation (caval, bowel)

5.3 SVC Obstruction

| Presentation | Characterized by cyanosis, and swelling of the head, neck and upper limbs |
| | Associated with orbital oedema, proptosis and venous distension |

Aetiology	Mediastinal neoplasms (primary bronchogenic, secondary or lymphoma) 90%
	Mediastinal fibrosis (secondary to aneurysmal dilatation of the aorta or right subclavian artery)
	Thrombosis secondary to central venous lines

Investigations	Chest X-ray
	CT
	Venography
	MR venography

Malignant SVC obstruction

Treatment options

Radiotherapy:
- slow response (approximately 1–2 weeks)
- response is complete in approximately 20% of patients, partial in 50%
- recurrence rate is in the range of 10–32%

Chemotherapy:
- indicated for small-cell carcinoma/lymphoma

Bypass surgery:
- patients frequently are not fit enough to undergo surgical intervention
- associated morbidity and mortality is high in patients with, in most cases, a short life span

Interventional therapy

Venous stenting is a simple and effective treatment that can be undertaken in patients unfit for surgery who are unable to wait for the response of either radiotherapy or chemotherapy

Patient preparation

Informed consent
Local anaesthetic only

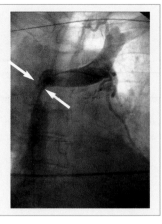

Figure 5.31
Venogram
demonstrating extrinsic
compression of the
SVC by tumour mass
(arrows)

Procedure

Bilateral venograms are performed to confirm the diagnosis and to allow visualization of the anatomy (Figure 5.31)

If thrombus is present, this may require thrombolysis prior to stent placement

The stenosis is traversed and measured prior to stent placement followed by a check venogram (Figure 5.32, 5.33)

Post-procedural formal anticoagulation is of debatable benefit

Figure 5.32
Expandable metal stent placed across SVC stenosis. Rapid flow through SVC into right atrium

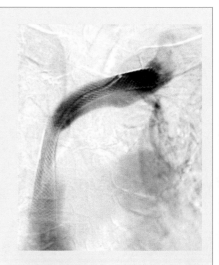

Figure 5.33
Unsubtracted image showing stent position

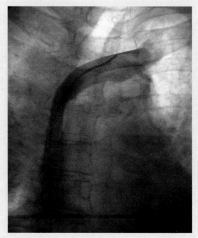

| Outcome | High technical success rate – patient selection is important |
| | Outcome appears to be better than with other techniques available, especially in the seriously ill patient |

| Complications | Stent migration/fracture |
| | Recurrent stenosis with tumour progression |

Benign SVC obstruction

| Treatment options | Surgical bypass should be considered although morbidity and mortality are high |

Interventional therapy	Can be used and balloon angioplasty is easy to perform
	Recurrence rates are high and stenting should be reserved for those with failed treatment
	Long-term patency is still not known

Arterial Intervention

Vascular intervention has developed from simple diagnostic angiography into a spectrum of procedures with increasing scope and complexity. This has resulted in endovascular therapy becoming the standard treatment in a large number of vascular cases. Interventional vascular radiology is generally associated with lower morbidity and mortality than standard surgical techniques. The development of an increasing range of wires, catheters, stents and therapeutic agents means that, in the future, even more vascular problems will be solved by the percutaneous route.

5.4 Percutaneous Transluminal Angioplasty (PTA)

This technique involves the balloon dilatation of a stenosis or occlusion within a blood vessel. The most common reason for vascular disease is atherosclerosis. Other disease entities such as trauma, fibromuscular dysplasia, intimal hyperplasia and connective tissue disorders can also be treated by PTA.

Indications

Lifestyle limiting claudication, unresponsive to conservative management or exercise

Critical ischaemia; rest pain, ulceration or tissue loss (limb salvage)

'Blue-toe syndrome' – microembolization resulting in painful cyanotic lesions within the distal lower limbs

Maintenance of graft patency – surveillance and secondary intervention can markedly improve the long-term patency of vascular grafts

Investigations

There is increasing usage of non-invasive imaging (Duplex and MRA) for the diagnosis and planning of intervention

Contraindications

Absolute

Recent thrombosis requiring treatment by thrombolysis ± aspiration

Relative

Bleeding diatheses (correct prior to treatment)

Patients with procoagulant states (vascular intervention is usually unsuccessful in this group)

Aortic and iliac occlusion (increasingly treated by primary stent deployment)

Patient preparation

Informed consent

Intravenous access

Aspirin therapy – should be started 48 h prior to intervention, unless contraindicated

Heparin – 5000 units given intra-arterially during the procedure

Antispasmodic agents (nifedipine 10–20 mg orally/glyceryl trinitrate 150–300 μg intra-arterially) – prevent arterial spasm during vessel manipulation

Procedure

Aseptic technique

Arterial access:

- can be single or double wall puncture depending upon the operator and the procedure to be performed; single wall punctures are advisable if thrombolysis is undertaken; double wall punctures are historically associated with fewer complications
- can be via antegrade or retrograde approach depending on site of obstruction (see Table 5.41)

Lower limb	Upper limb
Common femoral artery	Axillary artery
Superficial femoral artery	Brachial artery
Profunda femoris	Radial artery
Popliteal artery	
Bypass grafts (under antibiotic cover)	

Table 5.41 Access routes for PTA

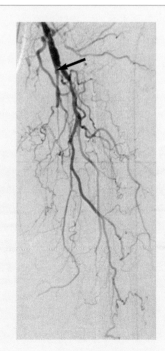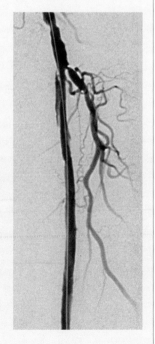

Figure 5.41
Occlusion of the left superficial femoral artery at the origin of profunda femoris (arrow). Extensive collateralization

Figure 5.42
Subintimal approach and balloon angioplasty with good flow within the SFA via an antegrade approach from the left common femoral artery

Arteriography is performed to confirm the lesion; this is then traversed by a standard/hydrophilic guidewire, supported by a catheter; distal vessel patency is then confirmed

Having traversed the lesion, the guidewire remains across the lesion

Balloon dilatation is performed – this allows fracturing of the atheromatous plaque and medial dissection (Figure 5.42)

The size of balloon selected depends on the diameter of the vessel and the length of the lesion

The balloon is usually inflated (using an inflation device/by hand) until the waisting disappears

Balloon dilatation results in pain that should be tolerable – if this is not the case, one should suspect either impending rupture or that the balloon may be subintimally placed within the vessel wall

This technique is standard within the intravascular system and has the advantage of being repeatable when necessary

Outcome

Technical success is high:

- iliac lesions — 90–95% for stenoses, less for occlusions
- femoral and popliteal artery lesions — 85–95% for stenoses, 60–90% for occlusions, with patency rates of 45–85% at 2 years
- Improved patency for occlusions using the sub-initimal technique

Definition of success is based on the absence of any residual pressure gradient across the lesion (this is only accurate within the aorto-iliac segments) and the angiographic appearance (no residual stenosis)

Further success can be measured by ABPI (ankle brachial pressure index) and intravascular ultrasound

Complications

Overall 2–3%

Puncture site	PTA site	Systemic circulation
Haematoma	Thrombus perforation	Septicaemia
Infection	Rupture pseudoaneurysm	Embolic occlusion
Dissection		Deterioration in renal function
Thrombosis		Cholesterol embolization
Pseudoaneurysm formation		
Arteriovenous fistula		

Table 5.42 Complications of PTA

Special case: **Renal angioplasty**

Renovascular hypertension is found in 4–5% of patients with hypertension caused by fibromuscular dysplasia (FMD) or atherosclerosis. FMD has good results and outcome with PTA. Atherosclerosis, particularly at the ostia, has good technical outcome with stent placement. The benefits following a technical success are still under investigation. The outcome in improving hypertension appears to be better than in preventing deteriorating renal function, although trials are currently being performed to improve patient selection

Presentation

Hypertension – poor control with medical management
Deteriorating renal function
(Renal transplant artery stenosis)

Investigations

Routine blood screens
Renal nuclear medicine scan – MAG3
Doppler ultrasound
Arteriography/MRA

Patient preparation

Informed consent
Intravenous access
Local anaesthetic ± sedation

Procedure

Standard femoral approach/brachial approach (if AAA [abdominal aortic aneurysm] or aortic occlusive atheromatous disease)
Confirmation of the renal artery lesion by a flush aortogram

Selective renal arteriography (Figure 5.43, 5.44)

Intra-arterial heparin (5000 IU) and GTN (glyceryl trinitrate)

The lesion is traversed using a hydrophilic guidewire, so allowing catheter advancement

A stiff guidewire is then placed across the lesion and balloon angioplasty is performed until the waist disappears

Figure 5.43
MRA demonstrating bilateral renal artery stenosis (arrows). Worse on the left

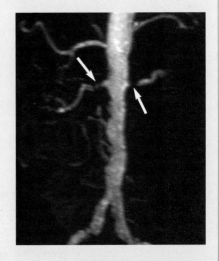

Figure 5.44
Digital subtraction angiography confirming bilateral renal artery stenosis (arrows)

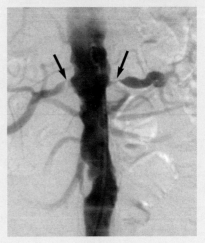

Figure 5.45
Angiographic
appearance following
bilateral angioplasty
and stent insertion
(arrows)

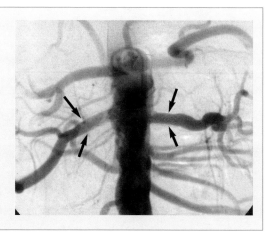

Figure 5.45
Angiographic
appearance following
bilateral angioplasty
and stent insertion
(arrows)

Technical success is confirmed by the absence of stenosis on post-dilatation arteriography

If the stenosis fails to dilate or if it recurs, a balloon-expandable stent can be used (ostial atheromata are treated by primary stent deployment in most centres) (Figure 5.45)

Outcome

Technical success rate:
- 90% for stenoses for PTA
- 50% for occlusions for PTA

For stent placement success rate approaches >95%

Long-term results:
- fibromuscular dysplasia – 90% show improvement of hypertension
- atheromatous disease – 60–70% show improved control of hypertension
- stabilization or improvement of renal function is still under investigation

Complications

Deterioration in renal function (5%)
Renal artery occlusion (3–4%)
Renal artery rupture (1%)

The significance of these complications and the risk of loss of viability to the kidney make it mandatory that vascular surgical support is present within the institution in which renal angioplasty/stent placement is being performed

5.5 Vascular Stents

Endovascular stents have been developed to support the arterial wall mechanically, so maintaining patency of the lumen

Indications

Stenoses with a persistent pressure gradient (aorto-iliac segments) following PTA
Acute occlusion caused by the formation of an intimal flap dissection following angioplasty
Iliac occlusions
Recurrent stenoses or a previous PTA site
Aneurysmal disease

To date, stents have mainly been used in aorto-iliac disease (Figures 5.51–5.54); however, they are becoming increasingly used in other sites, for example: renal ostial atheroma, subclavian and common carotid arteries

Figure 5.51
DSA illustrating occlusion of the left external iliac artery at its origin

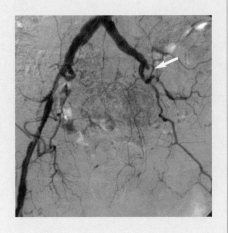

Figure 5.52
The lesion has been traversed and the stent placed across the stenosis

Figure 5.53
Stent deployment

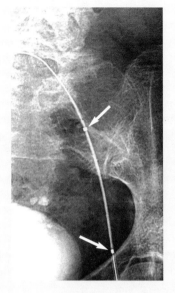
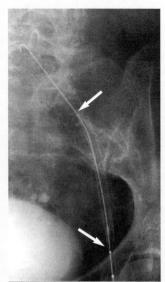

Figure 5.54
Post stent placement, good flow through the left external iliac into the common femoral artery

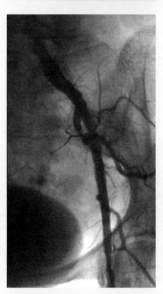

Outcome   Technical success rate 98–100%

Complications   As for PTA

Acute thrombosis

Stenosis secondary to intimal hyperplasia – this is not usually amenable to balloon dilatation and considerable research is being carried out to develop drugs and in intraluminal radiation in an attempt to limit in-stent restenosis

Special case:

Endovascular stenting of abdominal aortic aneursyms

Abdominal aortic aneurysms (AAA) remain a disease with a significant morbidity and mortality. There is a large variation of outcomes in both elective and emergency treatment of this patient group

The UK small aneurysm study has shown no benefit in the treatment of aneurysms between 4 cm and 5.5 cm. Aneurysms larger than this show an increased risk of symptomatic presentation and have been found positively to benefit from active management

Presentation

Asymptomatic – aneurysm identified at routine ultrasound or clinical examination

Symptomatic – rapid enlargement of the aneurysm
Development of periaortic inflammation
Leak
Rupture

Investigations

The elective setting:
Full blood count
Clot and screen
Cross-matching
Ultrasound
Contrast enhanced CT
Angiography

The emergency setting:
Full blood count

Clotting

Cross-matching

Imaging is dependent upon the haemodynamic stability of the patient

Treatment options

Surgery

Open repair is the traditional treatment for patients who are fit for surgery and has a low incidence of morbidity and mortality

In the case of ruptured aneurysms, even within specialist centres, morbidity and mortality remain high (approximately 50%)

However, endovascular repair is increasingly being performed in carefully selected cases after careful radiological evaluation

Interventional therapy

Endovascular techniques have been developed to provide a less invasive alternative to open surgery. The Eurostar database (a European prospective study) has confirmed the high degree of success in the deployment of aortic endografts with only low complication rates. The aneurysm needs to fulfill strict criteria to allow the use of endovascular stents. As a result, 30–40% of all AAAs are suitable for endovascular repair (Figure 5.53, 5.54)

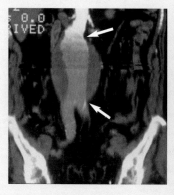 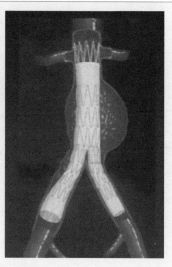

Figure 5.53
Intravenous contrast enhanced spiral CT (coronal reconstruction) showing infra renal aortic aneurysm

Figure 5.54
An endovascular AAA stent with bilateral iliac limbs

Patient preparation	Endovascular repair of abdominal aneurysms can be undertaken in either a radiological operating suite or main operating theatres under a general anaesthetic usually with vascular and radiological teams being present. High quality fluoroscopy and digital subtraction angiography is mandatory
Procedure	Dependent upon the type of endoprosthesis used Bilateral femoral arteriotomies are undertaken and diagnostic angiograms performed to allow visualization of the aneurysm The delivery system of the endoprosthesis is then advanced within the aorta until the top markers line up above the level of the renal arteries Graft deployment is then commenced and the graft positioned such that its upper limit lies just below the renal arteries The remainder of the graft is then deployed The remaining iliac limb is then inserted via the contralateral femoral artery. Once correct positioning is achieved this is deployed A contrast enhanced CT examination is performed prior to discharge from hospital to confirm successful exclusion of the aneurysm. Follow up CT is performed at regular intervals; 3/12, 6/12, 12/12 and then annually to ensure endoleak does not occur and the aneurysm is not increasing in size
Outcome	Technical success 98%
Complications	Technical problems 17% In-hospital mortality rate 2.5% Graft thrombosis Vessel damage Endoleak (early/late) Current studies confirm the high initial technical success rate of endovascular repair of abdominal aortic aneurysms with low

morbidity and mortality if strict selection criteria are adhered to, however, long-term durability of the procedure is still not proven. In the UK, two trials are in progress: EVAR I and EVAR II. In EVAR I patients suitable for endovascular and open surgical repair are randomized to either technique. In EVAR II patients unsuitable for open surgical repair but anatomically suitable for endovascular repair are randomized to endovascular repair or best medical treatment. Further developments in endovascular grafts in the future will allow their use in supra-renal, thoraco-abdominal aneurysms, thoracic aneurysms and dissections as well as increasing their use in the acutely presenting AAA leak or rupture.

5.6 Arterial Thrombolysis

Over recent years, patients with acute limb ischaemia caused by underlying longstanding atheromatous disease rather than by embolic occlusion have become increasingly common. The pathophysiology in these patients has meant that there is poor surgical outcome following embolectomy. This has resulted in an increased use of arterial thrombolysis.

It should be noted that thrombolysis alone will not cure these patients and that they ultimately need treatment of their underlying atheromatous disease. This may be by achieved by endovascular or surgical means.

Indications

Proximal/distal arterial thrombosis, especially with poor distal run-off

Distal arterial emboli – where surgical embolectomy would result in damage

Thrombosis of a venous or synthetic graft

Thrombosis at the site of previous vascular intervention

Contraindications

Absolute   Cerebrovascular accident (within 6 months), transient ischaemic attack (within 2 months)
Intracranial tumour
Active internal bleeding

Relative   Recent surgery within 10–14 days
Gastrointestinal bleeding
Trauma
Uncontrolled hypertension
Diabetic retinopathy

Presentation

History of intermittent claudication with associated risk factors (diabetes mellitus, hypercholesterolaemia, smoking, family history)

The limb is:
- painful
- pale
- perishingly cold
- paraesthetic
- pulseless

Patient selection is important. If there is irreversible ischaemia (increasing sensori-motor deficit with calf tenderness) thrombolysis is contraindicated

Investigations

Routine blood screens
ECG – to exclude atrial fibrillation as the source of possible thrombi
Colour Doppler ultrasound
Arteriography
MRA (Magnetic resonance angiography)

Interventional therapy

Patient preparation   Informed consent

Intravenous access

Local anaesthetic ± sedation

Opiate-based analgesia

Adequate fluid replacement

Intravenous heparin should be run concurrently during the thrombolysis and continued until any underlying lesion is treated

Antispasmodic drugs (glyceryl trinitrate – 150 μg given intravenously in 30–50 μg aliquots)

Procedure

Aseptic technique

A standard common femoral approach is usually performed from the contralateral limb

Diagnostic angiography is undertaken to confirm the presence of acute thrombosis (Figure 5.61a, 5.61b)

An intra-arterial catheter is placed within the thrombus of the occluded segment and, if feasible, a small catheter or an infusion line is placed distally at the level of the trifurcation

Thrombolysis is performed (Figure 5.61c, 5.61d)

There are two basic techniques for arterial thrombolysis:

- low-dose infusion
- pulse spray

In addition to thrombolysis, acute thrombosis can be treated by aspiration thromboembolectomy or mechanical thrombectomy

Outcome

Limb salvage rate 70–80%

Amputation rate 5–10%

Complications

Groin haematoma

Retroperitoneal haemorrhage

Peri-catheter thrombosis

Distal embolization

Acute renal failure

Cerebrovascular accident

Figure 5.61

a) Flush angiogram in a 59 year old man with an acutely ischaemic limb, showing occlusion of the right external iliac artery (arrow)

b) The right external iliac artery has been traversed and there is evidence of thrombus within it (arrow)

c) Thrombolysis is performed and at check angiography at 16 h the flow is considerably improved. Note the internal iliac artery has recanalized

d) At 18 h the thrombus has almost completely dissolved and good flow is re-established

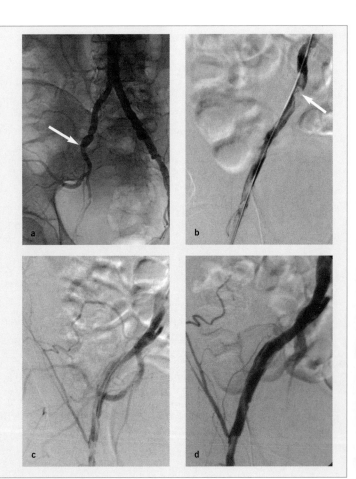

5.7 Embolization

Embolization is the deliberate occlusion of blood vessels or vascular spaces by embolic material.

The technique is used in both emergency and elective settings. It requires a good understanding of arterial anatomy, the ability to undertake superselective catheterization and, in case of complications, full surgical cover.

Indications	Trauma:
	• haemorrhage (Figures 5.71–5.74)
	• AV fistulae
	Arteriovenous malformations:
	• definitive treatment – preoperative reduction in the size and vascularity of the malformation
	• palliative management – to reduce symptomatology
	Tumours:
	• definitive management of benign lesions – preoperative reduction in the size and vascularity of the lesion, so allowing surgical resection
	• palliative management – to reduce symptomatology
Contraindications	
Absolute	None
Relative	In cases where the arterial supply is from end arteries, so increasing the risk of ischaemia and possible necrosis (e.g. the gastrointestinal tract, beyond the duodenojejunal flexure, carries a significant risk of infarction of the gut)
Treatment options	
Surgery	Dependent upon the site but usually carries significant morbidity and mortality – this is significantly reduced if preoperative embolization is undertaken
Interventional therapy	
Patient preparation	Informed consent
	Intravenous access
	Adequate analgesia
	Antibiotic cover

Procedure   Standard angiography (using digital subtraction) is performed
                 to allow a detailed 'road map' of the local arterial anatomy
                 Superselective catheterization is necessary to avoid the inadvertent

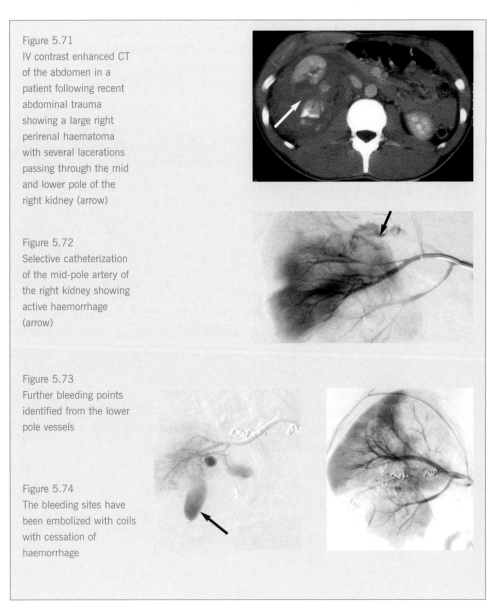

Figure 5.71
IV contrast enhanced CT
of the abdomen in a
patient following recent
abdominal trauma
showing a large right
perirenal haematoma
with several lacerations
passing through the mid
and lower pole of the
right kidney (arrow)

Figure 5.72
Selective catheterization
of the mid-pole artery of
the right kidney showing
active haemorrhage
(arrow)

Figure 5.73
Further bleeding points
identified from the lower
pole vessels

Figure 5.74
The bleeding sites have
been embolized with coils
with cessation of
haemorrhage

embolization of surrounding arterial branches – this also ensures
that the embolic agent is delivered to the nidus of the lesion,
so improving the chances of its complete obliteration (Figure 5.72)
Various types of embolic materials are available – the choice
depends upon both the site and the nature of the area to
be embolized

When embolizing an area, it is essential to occlude all potential
feeders – otherwise, filling of the lesion may occur by retrograde flow,
which will ultimately lead to failure of the treatment (Figure 5.73)

Nature	Embolic material	Occlusion
Trauma	Sterile absorbable gelatine sponge, PVA particles/coils	Temporary/permanent
Haemorrhage	PVA particles/coils	Semi-permanent
Tumour	Particles	Semi-permanent
Arteriovenous malformations	Coils/alcohol/glue	Permanent
	Detachable balloons	Permanent
Aneurysms	Sclerosing agents (isobutyl-2-cyanoacrylate)	Permanent
	Coils	Permanent
	Detachable balloons	Permanent

Table 5.71 Types of embolic agents and indications for their use

Outcome

Technical success varies depending upon the site and nature of the
area to be embolized but is improving with better catheter design
and trackability. Usually better for fistula and aneurysms rather
than malformations

Complications

Post-embolization syndrome – this is common and consists of
malaise, pyrexia, pain and leucocytosis, which can persist for up
to 5 days post treatment; these symptoms increase with an
increase in the volume of tissue embolized; necessitates the use of
systemic antibiotic therapy

Excessive tissue necrosis – process of embolization results in
controlled necrosis; however, if a large area is infarcted, this can
lead to significant ischaemia with subsequent manifestations

Inadvertent embolization of normal structures – this can be caused by an unstable catheter position or inadequate selectivity of the arterial supply

Pulmonary embolization – particulate embolic material can occasionally pass through arteriovenous communications and ultimately become lodged within the pulmonary circulation; when this does occur, conservative treatment is usually adequate

This is best avoided by not using particulate in AVMs

ARTERIAL EMBOLIZATION

What is arterial embolization?

The doctors have discovered that you have an artery that needs to be deliberately blocked off. This may be the result of uncontrollable bleeding or be an abnormal blood supply to a specific organ or area. In order to stop the blood flow through this artery, special particles, glue or tiny wire coils must be placed in the vessel.

What happens?

In order for the abnormal artery to be seen and the site of embolization accurately localized, an angiogram is performed (you may wish to read the section on femoral angiograms). A catheter (tube) is then manoeuvred so that it lies within the vessel to be embolized. The radiologist then carefully introduces the 'glue' or stainless steel coils until no further blood flow is seen in the vessel. You will have an X-ray camera over your abdomen so that the radiologist can see the tube. The radiologist will ask you to keep very still as he takes some X-ray pictures; he may also ask you to hold your breath for a few seconds. The X-ray contrast may make you feel quite warm; however, this is normal and doesn't last very long.

How long will it take?

The actual procedure usually takes about 1 h although you should expect to be in the department for about 2 h.

Is it painful?

This depends on the site being embolized. If necessary, you can have a sedative and painkilling injection via a vein in your hand. This will make you sleepy and free of discomfort, but will still allow you to co-operate during the procedure.

Afterwards

When the radiologist is satisfied that the vessel has been completely blocked and the blood flow stopped, the catheter will be removed and you will need to stay on bed rest for 6 h. The nurse will check your pulse and blood pressure at regular intervals and will also check your groin for signs of bleeding. You will be given strong painkillers to ease the pain, if necessary. It is usual in the following few days to experience mild fever and you may experience 'flu-like' symptoms.

CENTRAL VENOUS ACCESS LINES (HICKMANN/TESSIO LINE INSERTION)

What is a central venous access line?

This is an X-ray examination whereby a special tube (or line) is placed within the heart via a vein in the neck.

Preparation

The nurses on the ward will help you to get ready. You must not eat for 2 h before the procedure, and a doctor on the ward will explain the procedure to you so that you can sign a consent form. Please ask any questions you wish. You may have your skin (neck and shoulders) washed with a special soap and be given some antibiotics to prevent infection during the examination.

What happens?

The outer end of a special tube or line is 'tunnelled' on to the chest, to help reduce the risk of infection. This line enables easy and quick administration of drugs into the body without the use of needles. The central venous access or Hickman lines are used for the administration of special feeds or chemotherapy drugs, and Tessio lines are used for venous dialysis in renal patients.

How long will it take?

The procedure is normally completed within an hour.

Is it painful?

In the X-ray department you will be expected to lie flat on your back on an X-ray table.

You will be given oxygen and can have a sedative injection via a vein in your hand. This will make you sleepy, but will still allow you to co-operate during the procedure.

An injection of local anaesthetic is given into the skin of the neck. This will sting initially but will quickly make the area go numb.

You will now only be aware of a pushing sensation as the line is moved into position. The X-ray machine is used to check that the lines are in the correct position and this will be moved around you during the procedure.

Afterwards

When the procedure is finished, a dressing will be placed over the wound and you will need to stay in bed for a few hours. During this time a nurse will take regular checks of your pulse and blood pressure.

Results

The line will be in the correct place when you leave the department as it has been checked using X-rays during the procedure.

INFERIOR VENA CAVA FILTER INSERTION

What is an IVC filter?

You will probably already have had a CT, ultrasound or venogram (an injection of dye into the veins in the back of foot) and the doctors have discovered clots affecting your legs. These clots can break off and block the arteries supplying the lungs. One way of preventing this is to put a filter (sieve) in the main vein in your abdomen. This traps the clots from the legs and stops them getting to the lungs.

Preparation

A doctor on the ward will explain the procedure to you and ask you to sign a consent form. If you suffer from asthma, hayfever or have any allergies you must inform the doctor or nurse who is looking after you. On the day of the procedure the nurses on the ward will ensure that you are properly prepared. They will ask you to shave both sides of the groin and change into a hospital gown. You should also have nothing to eat or drink 2 h before the examination. Once in the X-ray department, an X-ray nurse will greet you and check that you have been properly prepared.

What happens?

The radiologist (X-ray doctor) then inserts a small tube (catheter) into your femoral vein (at the top of your leg) or internal jugular vein (in the neck). You will have an X-ray camera over your abdomen so that the radiologist can see the tube. Some contrast is injected into the tube and this will flow into the veins in your abdomen. The radiologist will ask you to keep very still as he takes some X-ray pictures; he/she may also ask you to hold your breath for a few seconds. The X-ray contrast may make you feel quite warm; however, this is normal and doesn't last very long. Having identified the exact position of the leg clots and the inferior vena cava (main vein), the radiologist will then insert the filter via the tube in your groin or neck. This usually will not hurt. Finally, some X-rays are taken to check the position of the filter in your vein.

Is it painful?

In the X-ray department you will be expected to lie flat on your back on an X-ray table. If you are having difficulty breathing we can raise you on the table and give you oxygen.

An injection of local anaesthetic is given into the skin of the groin or neck. This will sting initially but will quickly make the area go numb.

How long will it take?

The actual procedure usually takes about 45 minutes although you should expect to be in the department for about an hour.

Afterwards

You will be asked not to bend your leg for a few hours afterwards. This is to ensure the puncture sight does not bleed. Once back on the ward you will have to remain in bed for about 6 h afterwards. The nurse will check your pulse and blood pressure at regular intervals and will also check your groin for signs of bleeding. You may eat and drink normally.

Results

Your doctors will be contacted with regards to the procedure and further treatment needed.

SUPERIOR VENA CAVA STENT INSERTION

What is an SVC stent? You will probably already have had a CT or venogram (an injection of dye into the veins in the back of both your hands) and the doctors have discovered a narrowing of the superior vena cava (the large vein in your chest draining into your heart). One way of treating this, is to stretch the vein with a balloon and use a stent (spring) to keep it open. This will help the blood flow more easily through the vein and should rapidly improve your symptoms.

Preparation A doctor on the ward will explain the procedure to you and ask you to sign a consent form. If you suffer from asthma, hayfever or have any allergies you must inform the doctor or nurse who is looking after you. On the day of the procedure the nurses on the ward will ensure that you are properly prepared. They will ask you to shave both sides of the groin and change into a hospital gown. You should also have nothing to eat or drink 2 h before the examination. Once in the X-ray department, you will be greeted by an X-ray nurse, who will check that you have been properly prepared.

What happens? The radiologist (X-ray doctor) inserts a small tube (catheter) into your femoral vein (at the top of your leg). You will have an X-ray camera over your chest so that the radiologist can see the tube. Some contrast is injected into the tube and this will flow into the veins in your chest. The radiologist will ask you to keep very still as he/she takes some X-ray pictures; he/she may also ask you to hold your breath for a few seconds. The X-ray contrast may make you feel quite warm; however, this is normal and doesn't last very long. Having identified the exact position of the narrowing, the radiologist will then insert the stent via the tube in your groin. This will not hurt. Finally, some X-rays are taken to see the blood flowing through the stent in your vein and into the heart.

How long will it take?   The actual procedure usually takes about 45 minutes although you should expect to be in the department for about an hour.

Is it painful?   In the X-ray department you will be expected to lie flat on your back on an X-ray table. If you are having difficulty breathing you will be raised on the table and given oxygen.
An injection of local anaesthetic is given into the skin of the groin. This will sting initially but will quickly make the area go numb.

Afterwards   You will be asked not to bend your leg for a few hours afterwards. This is to ensure the puncture sight does not bleed. Once back on the ward you will have to remain in bed for about 6 h afterwards. The nurse will check your pulse and blood pressure at regular intervals and will also check your groin for signs of bleeding. You may eat and drink normally.

Results   You should notice a rapid improvement in your symptoms over the next few days.

FEMORAL ANGIOGRAM

What is a femoral angiogram?

This is an X-ray examination of the arteries in your legs. On a normal X-ray the blood vessels are not easily seen, so the radiologist (X-ray doctor) needs to inject a dye (contrast) into the blood vessels so that they can be visualized. Once the contrast is in the blood vessels the radiologist will take some X-rays and study them carefully after the examination.

Preparation

A doctor on the ward will explain the procedure to you and ask you to sign a consent form. This usually happens the day before the examination. If you suffer from asthma, hayfever or have any allergies you must inform the doctor or nurse who is looking after you. On the day of the procedure the nurses on the ward will ensure that you are properly prepared. They will ask you to shave your groin and change into a hospital gown. You should also have nothing to eat or drink 2 h before the examination. Once in the X-ray department, you will be greeted by an X-ray nurse, who will check that you have been properly prepared.

What happens?

You will lie on the X-ray table and the radiologist will clean your groin area with some cleaning solution. He/she will then cover you with a sterile drape. It is important that things remain sterile so you need to keep your hands by your side during the whole procedure. The radiologist inserts a small tube (catheter) into your femoral artery (at the top of your leg). You will have an X-ray camera over your abdomen so that the radiologist can see the tube. Some contrast is injected into the tube and this will flow into the arteries in your legs. The radiologist will ask you to keep very still as he takes some X-ray pictures; he/she may also ask you to hold your breath for a few seconds. The X-ray contrast may make you feel quite warm; however, this is normal and doesn't last very long. A series of pictures will be taken all the way down your legs so that all the arteries can be seen. The tube will then be removed and the radiologist will press on your groin for a few minutes.

How long will it take?

The actual procedure usually takes about 30 minutes although you should expect to be in the department for about an hour.

Is it painful?

The radiologist will inject some local anaesthetic into the skin of your groin. The area will quickly become numb so you shouldn't feel any pain.

Afterwards

You will be asked not to bend your leg for a few hours afterwards. This is to ensure the puncture sight does not bleed. Once back on the ward you will have to remain in bed for about 6 h afterwards and lie flat for 4 h. The nurse will check your pulse and blood pressure at regular intervals and will also check your groin for signs of bleeding. You may eat and drink normally. This is being increasingly performed as a daycase procedure. If the procedure has been performed in the morning you should be able to go home that evening or the following day.

Results

The results will reach the doctors within 24 h. The doctor will usually discuss the results with you in a follow up clinic, when the radiologist may or may not be present.

ANGIOPLASTY

What is an angioplasty?

You will probably already have had vascular studies (non-invasive or angiography, if not please read the section on angiograms) and the doctors have discovered a narrowing of one of your arteries. One way of treating this is to stretch the artery with a balloon. This will help the blood flow more easily through the artery. This technique is called an angioplasty.

Preparation

A doctor on the ward will explain the procedure to you and ask you to sign a consent form. Please ask any questions you wish. This usually happens the day before the examination. If you suffer from asthma, hayfever or have any allergies you must inform the doctors or nurses who are looking after you. On the day of the procedure the nurses on the ward will ensure that you are properly prepared. They will ask you to shave both sides of the groin and change into a hospital gown. You should also have nothing to eat or drink 2 h before the examination. The X-ray porter will collect you and wheel you down on your bed accompanied by a ward nurse. Once in the X-ray department you will be greeted by an X-ray nurse who will check that you have been properly prepared.

What happens?

You will lie on the X-ray table and the radiologist will clean your groin area with some cleaning solution. He/she will then cover you with a sterile drape. It is important that things remain sterile so you need to keep your hands by your side during the whole procedure. The radiologist will then inject some local anaesthetic into the skin of your groin. After a small stinging sensation, the area will quickly become numb, so you shouldn't feel any pain. The radiologist then inserts a small tube (catheter, usually into your femoral artery). You will have an X-ray camera over your abdomen so that the radiologist can see the tube. Some contrast is injected into the tube and this will show the narrowing in the artery. The narrowing is then stretched with the balloon. The radiologist will ask you to keep very still as he\she takes some X-ray pictures. The X-ray contrast may make you feel quite warm; however, this is normal and doesn't last very long.

When the radiologist has taken all the X-rays he/she needs, the tube will then be removed and the radiologist will press on your groin for a few minutes.

How long will it take? The actual procedure usually takes about 30 minutes although you should expect to be in the department for about an hour.

Is it painful? There is only minor discomfort when the vessel is stretched. If you feel anxious about this, you can have a sedative injection via a vein in your hand. This will make you sleepy, but will still allow you to co-operate during the procedure.

Afterwards You will be asked not to bend your leg or sit up for 4 h afterwards. This is to ensure the puncture site does not bleed. Once back on the ward you will have to remain in bed for about 6 h afterwards and lie flat for 2 h. The nurse will check your pulse and blood pressure at regular intervals and will also check your groin for signs of bleeding. You may eat and drink normally. If the procedure is performed in the morning you may be allowed home that evening or the following day.

Results On your return to the ward, follow-up and future management can be arranged.

VASCULAR STENT INSERTION

What is a stent insertion?

You will probably already have had vascular studies (non-invasive or angioplasty, if not please read the section on angiograms) and the doctor has decided to place a stent inside your artery to help the blood flow more easily through it. The stent is a kind of 'spring' made of metal that holds open the artery. The stent will remain there permanently but you won't notice it is there. It should help greatly improve your symptoms.

Preparation

A doctor on the ward will explain the procedure to you and ask you to sign a consent form. This usually happens the day before the examination. If you suffer from asthma or hayfever, have any allergies or are diabetic you must inform the doctor or nurse who is looking after you. On the day of the procedure the nurses on the ward will ensure that you are properly prepared. They will ask you to shave both sides of the groin and change into a hospital gown. You should also have nothing to eat or drink 2 h before the examination. In the X-ray department you will be greeted by an X-ray nurse who will check that you have been properly prepared.

What happens?

You will lie on the X-ray table and the radiologist (X-ray doctor) will clean your groin area with some cleaning solution. He/she will then cover you with a sterile drape. It is important that things remain sterile so you need to keep your hands by your side during the whole procedure. The radiologist then inserts a small tube (catheter, usually into your femoral artery). You will have an X-ray camera over your abdomen so that the radiologist can see the tube. Some contrast is injected into the tube and this will flow into the artery where the stent is going to be placed. The radiologist will ask you to keep very still as he/she takes some X-ray pictures; he/she may also ask you to hold your breath for a few seconds. The X-ray contrast may make you feel quite warm; however, this is normal and doesn't last very long. A series of pictures will be taken of the narrowed artery. The radiologist will then insert the stent (expandable spring) via the tube (catheter) in your femoral artery. Finally, some X-rays are taken to see the blood flowing through the stent in your artery.

How long will it take?   The actual procedure usually takes about 1 h
although you should expect to be in the department for about 2 h.

Is it painful?   The radiologist will then inject some local anaesthetic into the skin of your groin. The area will quickly become numb so you shouldn't feel any pain.

Afterwards   You will be asked not to bend your leg for a few hours afterwards. This is to ensure the puncture site does not bleed. Once back on the ward you will have to remain in bed for about 6 h afterwards and lie flat for 2 h. The nurse will check your pulse and blood pressure at regular intervals and will also check your groin for signs of bleeding. You may eat and drink normally.

Results   The doctors will tell you the results when they have received them from the radiologist, and future follow-up can be arranged. Although, the radiologist will usually inform you and the attending ward nurse of the results and outcome immediately after the procedure.

ARTERIAL THROMBOLYSIS

What is thrombolysis?

The doctors have discovered that you have a blood clot (thrombus) in one of your arteries. In order for the blood to flow normally again the clot has to be dissolved. To do this a drug called tissue Plasminogen Activator (tPA) or urokinase can be administered onto or near the clot until it has dissolved completely and your blood flow is back to normal. These are powerful drugs and carry risks of causing bleeding anywhere in the body – in the abdomen, head (stroke) and from the groin.

What happens?

In order for a clot to be discovered, an angiogram is performed (you may wish to read the section on femoral angiograms). If a clot is discovered during the angiogram the radiologist (X-ray doctor) will call your consultant and decide whether tPA is the best treatment. They will of course discuss this with you. If thrombolysis is the treatment of choice, a longer catheter will be guided under X-ray control directly onto the clot or to an area close to it. Once the catheter has been secured firmly in place the tPA will be started. The tPA will be given to you added in 1 or 2 bags of fluid. These are attached to your catheter with a fluid bag and run through pumps to ensure a precise dose is given.

During thrombolysis you must not move the affected limb – in case of dislodging the catheter. You must also remain fairly flat and you will have to use a bedpan during the treatment. This will continue until the treatment is complete and for a further 12 h afterwards. This may sound very daunting and frightening but these precautions are carried out to ensure that you are kept as comfortable as possible.

How long will it take?   The treatment may last between 3 h and 3 days. During this time you will be closely monitored both on the ward and in the X-ray department. Every few hours, check angiograms will be carried out to see how much of the clot has dissolved. You will be kept fully informed at all times.

Is it painful?   tPA is a very powerful and effective drug; it is used with great care and with careful consideration. The very fact that it is so effective can cause side effects. Pain is fairly common but it maybe a good sign that the tPA is working. You will be given strong painkillers to ease the pain.

Afterwards   The nurse on the ward will check the puncture site in your groin at regular intervals. If you notice any bleeding please inform the nurses on the ward immediately. When the radiologist is satisfied that the clot has completely dissolved, the catheter will be removed and you will need to stay on bed rest for approximately 12 h.

Results   Depending on the effectiveness of the tPA therapy, there are a variety of further treatments. Your doctor will discuss these with you.

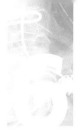

GYNAECOLOGICAL INTERVENTION

6.1 Post-partum Haemorrhage/Obstetric Haemorrhage

Presentation

Traditionally, obstetric haemorrhage – either anticipated or presenting as an emergency – has been treated by surgical means. Initially, this involves local control by means of a ligation or packing of bleeding sites. If this fails, hysterectomy is normally undertaken.

Obstetric patients can be divided into two groups:

- Those patients with antepartum or preoperative risk of bleeding (placenta accreta and praevia)
- Those with an expected post-partum/post-caesarean-section haemorrhage (uterine atony, placenta praevia and accreta, retained products, uterine or vaginal lacerations)

Investigations

In the emergency setting:
- Full blood count
- Clotting screen
- Cross-matching

Treatment options

- Ligation of the uterine arteries/local packing
- Emergency hysterectomy

Interventional therapy

Patient preparation

Intravenous access

Adequate resuscitation

Appropriate anaesthetic

Oxygen

1. Emergency group

Procedure

A common femoral approach is performed

Following this, flush aortography is undertaken to provide an 'arterial roadmap', so aiding selective catheterization (Figure 6.11)

Elective diagnostic angiography is then performed, with imaging of the internal pudendal, uterine and vaginal vessels

Embolization is undertaken on the basis of the demonstration of active/continuing haemorrhage (Figure 6.12, 6.13)

A variety of embolization agents can be used – particulate, gelatine sponge pledgets, glue or coils

Clinically, the endpoint is cessation of serious bleeding; radiographically, therapy is deemed successful when no further extravasation of contrast can be seen

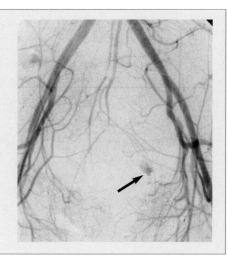

Figure 6.11
Flush aortogram reveals extravasation of contrast from a branch of the left uterine artery

Figure 6.12
Selective catheterization
of the left uterine artery.
Site of bleeding again
visualized

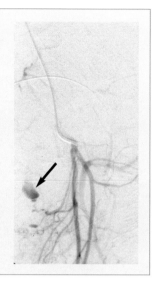

Outcome

This technique is being increasingly utilized, with several case series beginning to appear in the literature

Technical success rate is high

Complications

None significant

Normal menses are usually resumed after embolic therapy

Figure 6.13
Coils have been placed in
a distal branch of the
left uterine artery (arrow),
with subsequent
cessation of haemorrhage.
Non-subtracted image

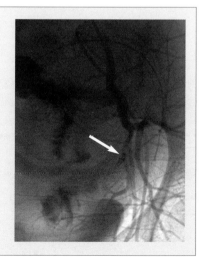

2. Prophylactic group

Procedure

Where indicated, interventional radiology may be undertaken prior to caesarean section

The gravid uterus is shielded with a lead apron

A brachial/axillary approach is preferred, as access is difficult within the patient's groin

Flush angiography is again performed and an 'arterial roadmap' produced

The catheter is left in situ at the level of the first lumbar vertebra

The patient is then transferred to the operating theatre for elective caesarean section

If, following the caesarean section, there is significant haemorrhage that is not controlled by local measures, the catheter can be advanced and selective catheterization and embolization performed as in the emergency group

6.2 Vulval Varices/Ovarian Vein Varices

Presentation

Chronic non-remitting pelvic pain, worsened by long periods of standing

Often associated with labial varices and varicose veins

Frequent association with dyspareunia

May also be found in asymptomatic women

Incidence within the UK female population: 5%

Investigations

Full gynaecological examination

Pelvic ultrasound

Laparoscopy

The exclusion of synchronous pathologies – pelvic inflammatory disease, endometriosis, neoplasia

Selective venography – via the left renal vein – to confirm the diagnosis of reflux into dilated ovarian veins

Treatment options

Surgical ligation

Successful in 73% of cases

Interventional therapy	Suitable for women with proven varicocoeles and conventional anatomy
	Embolization of ovarian varicocoeles can be done at the same time as the initial venography (single visit)
Contraindications	Co-existing pelvic pathology
	Aberrant venous anatomy
Patient preparation	Informed consent
	Appropriate analgesia ± sedation
Procedure	Aseptic technique
	Venous access is gained via the right or left femoral vein (Figure 6.21)
	A left renal venogram is performed to allow confirmation of the presence of reflux
	Coil embolization of ovarian veins (Figure 6.22, 6.23)
Outcome	Success rate 72%
Complications	Coil migration

Figure 6.21
Selective catheterization
of the left ovarian vein
showing variceal
dilatation (arrow)

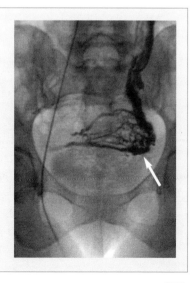

Figure 6.22
Embolization coils placed
within the left ovarian
vein, resulting in reduced
flow (arrows)

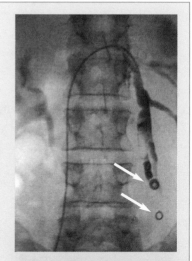

Figure 6.23
Occlusion of flow
within the left ovarian
vein. No filling of
varices

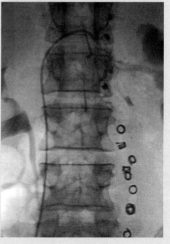

6.3 Fibroid Embolization

Presentation

Uterine fibroids (leiomyomas) are the most common tumour
in the female reproductive system

They commonly present with dysmenorrhoea and menorrhagia,
although occasionally can produce a mass effect and result in
urinary symptoms and focal neurology (sciatica)

Occur in 40% of women who are still menstruating at the age of 50
Increase in size and frequency with age, and are of increased
incidence among Afro-Caribbean women and nulliparous females

Investigations

Ultrasound
MRI (Figure 6.31)

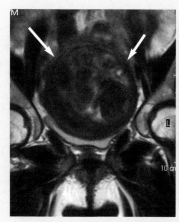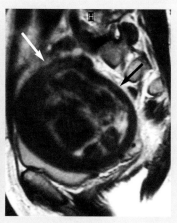

Figure 6.31
MRI showing enlarged
heterogeneous uterus
measuring 12 x 12 cm
(a) coronal section
(b) sagittal section

Treatment options

Hysterectomy –
abdominal/vaginal

Major operation requiring hospital stay of approximately 1 week,
with a long convalescence period

Myomectomy

The 'scooping out' of fibroids from the uterine wall
Can be performed abdominally or laparoscopically
Time-consuming and has a significant risk of haemorrhage

Medical management

Gonadatrophin-releasing-hormone analogues
Drug-induced shrinkage of the fibroids, but associated with side
effects and recurrence of the fibroid once treatment is finished

Interventional therapy

Has grown out of the desire among women not to undergo uterine
removal and to seek alternative therapies that allow organ
conservation – this is most marked among Afro-Caribbean women,

who culturally are very reluctant to undergo hysterectomy

The technique is still deemed experimental and full patient counselling is necessary before offering treatment

Indications

Dysmenorrhoea

Menorrhagia

Pressure related symptoms

Cycle related back pain

Frequency and nocturia

This procedure is not advised for asymptomatic fibroids or infertility

Patient preparation

Prior counselling – warning of the severe pain immediately following the procedure and then milder pain for several days subsequently

The discussions should include the risks of emergency hysterectomy (1–2%) and premature menopause (~1%)

Informed consent

Full blood count

Clotting screen

Close involvement of the gynaecological team and pain-control team – allowing the setting up of a patient-controlled analgesia (PCA) pump and providing sufficient back up immediately and in the follow up period

Procedure

A common femoral approach is performed

Selective catheterization of both internal iliacs with subselective catheterization of the uterine arteries is undertaken – this allows catheter placement to be secure and prevents any reflux when embolizing (Figure 6.32)

Embolization aims to effect the complete occlusion of both uterine arteries and is normally undertaken using medium-sized (300–500 microns) PVA (polyvinyl alcohol particles) (Figure 6.33)

The procedure is deemed technically successful if there is complete occlusion of both arteries

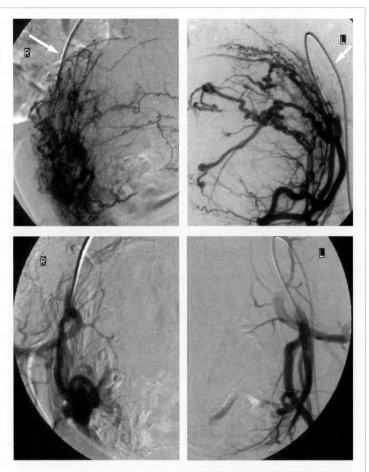

Figure 6.32
Digital subtraction
angiography of the left
and right internal
iliac arteries
pre-embolization
selective
catheterization of both
uterine arteries
(arrows)

Figure 6.33
Both uterine arteries
have been occluded
using particles

Outcome

95–100% technical success rate

~90% resolution of dysmenorrhoea, menorrhagia, urinary related
symptoms and back pain

Complications

Pain – this can be initially very severe, lasting for 12–18 h, and
often requires opiate suppression; a pain-relief protocol needs to
be devised

Post-embolization syndrome – fever, malaise, raised white count

Intermittent discharge

Spontaneous extrusion of fibroids per vaginum

Infection

Emergency hysterectomy 1-2%

Premature menopause ~1%

Follow-up, in the form of MRI scans at 3 months, 6 months and 1 year, is advised, to look at the extent of the necrosis and the volume reduction of the fibroid (normally 40–75%)

VARICEAL EMBOLIZATION

What is variceal embolization?

The doctors have discovered that you have an enlarged vein that needs to be deliberately blocked off. This may be the result of an abnormal blood supply to a specific organ or area. In order to stop the blood flow through this vein, tiny wire coils must be placed in the vessel. Other agents, sclerosants may also be used in order to achieve this.

What happens?

In order for the abnormal vein to be seen and the site of embolization accurately localized, a venogram is performed via a vein in the neck or groin (X-ray dye is injected using a catheter, introduced following a local anaesthetic injection). A catheter (tube) is then manoeuvred so that it lies within the vessel to be embolized. The radiologist then carefully introduces the stainless steel coils until no further blood flow is seen in the vessel. You will have an X-ray camera over your abdomen so that the radiologist can see the tube. The radiologist will ask you to keep very still as he takes some X-ray pictures; he may also ask you to hold your breath for a few seconds. The X-ray contrast (dye) may make you feel quite warm; however, this is normal and doesn't last very long.

Is it painful?

This depends on the site being embolized. If necessary, you can have a sedative and painkilling injection via a vein in your hand. This will make you sleepy and free of discomfort, but will still allow you to co-operate during the procedure.

How long does it take?

The actual procedure usually takes about 1 h although you should expect to be in the department for about 2 h.

Afterwards

When the radiologist is satisfied that the vessel has been completely blocked and the blood flow stopped, the catheter will be removed and you will need to stay on bed rest for 6 h. The nurse will check your pulse and blood pressure at regular intervals and will also check your groin for signs of bleeding. You will be given strong painkillers to ease the pain, if necessary.

FIBROID EMBOLIZATION

What is fibroid embolization?

The doctors have discovered that you have an enlarged uterus due to fibroids. An experimental treatment option is the deliberate blocking of the uterine arteries feeding the fibroids, so reducing their size, but preserving the uterus. In order to stop the blood flow through the fibroids, special 'glue' made of polyvinyl particles can be placed accurately in the uterine arteries.

Preparation

The radiologist will explain the procedure to you either in a clinic or on the ward. He/she will ask you to sign a consent form prior to the procedure in order that you can make the decision to proceed. On the day of the procedure the nurses on the ward will ensure that you are properly prepared. They will ask you to shave your groin and change into a hospital gown. You should also have nothing to eat or drink 2 h before the examination.

A member of the pain control team (anaesthetist or nurse) will come and see you on the ward and discuss their role in controlling the pain you may experience following the embolization. In the X-ray department, an X-ray nurse, who will check that you have been properly prepared, will greet you.

What happens?

In order for the uterine arteries to be seen and the site of embolization accurately localized an angiogram is performed (you may wish to read the section on femoral angiograms). A catheter (tube) is then manoeuvred so that it lies within the vessel to be embolized. The radiologist then carefully introduces the particles until no further blood flow is seen in both arteries. You will have an X-ray camera over your abdomen so that the radiologist can see the tube. The radiologist will ask you to keep very still as he/she takes some X-ray pictures; he/she may also ask you to hold your breath for a few seconds. The X-ray contrast may make you feel quite warm; however, this is normal and doesn't last very long.

How long will it take? The actual procedure usually takes about 1 h although you should expect to be in the department for about 2 h.

Is it painful? It can be painful, although the degree of discomfort varies from individual to individual. The pain usually starts immediately following the embolization. As described above, any pain you have will be dealt with promptly by the involvement of the pain relief team.

If you feel anxious, you can have a sedative and painkilling injection via a vein in your hand. This will make you sleepy and free of discomfort, but will still allow you to co-operate during the procedure.

Afterwards When the radiologist is satisfied that the vessel has been completely blocked and the blood flow stopped, the catheter will be removed and you will need to stay on bed rest for 6 h. The nurse will check your pulse and blood pressure at regular intervals and will also check your groin for signs of bleeding. You will be given strong painkillers to ease the pain, as necessary.

Prior to discharge, both the gynaecologists and the radiologist will see you.

Pain usually persists for 1 week following the embolization, but this is normally effectively managed with painkillers.

It is common to have a non-offensive vaginal discharge for some time. In addition, you may pass clots and solid material for several weeks.

As a result of the embolization, many patients have a fever and flu-like symptoms for several days. If this persists for more than 10 days or increases in severity, you should contact the gynaecologist or radiologist immediately. If you develop increasing pain, fever, chills, or lower abdominal tenderness with cramp-like pains, please contact your GP, radiologist or gynaecologist immediately.

INFERTILITY

7.1 Tubal Recanalization

Presentation

Approximately 30–40% of women with infertility have fallopian tube disease

Fallopian tube obstruction can be idiopathic or secondary to infection, tubal polyp, salpingitis, isthmica nodosa, endometriosis or congenital abnormalities

Investigations

Full gynaecological examination

Laparoscopy

Selective salpingography – to confirm the diagnosis and to exclude those individuals with spasm or transient obstruction

Treatment options

Tubal microsurgery and IVF – standard treatment option with an overall pregnancy rate of 28%

Interventional therapy

Suitable individuals are those with proven fallopian tube obstruction affecting the proximal segment of the tube (25% of women with tubal disease)

In this group, fallopian tube recanalization is now an accepted initial treatment

Contraindications

Distal tubal obstruction

Contrast allergy

Patient preparation	Informed consent
	Appropriate analgesia ± sedation
	Pre-procedural antibiotics – full 5-day course of antibiotics should follow the procedure

Procedure	Aseptic technique
	Selective salpingography using a 5.5 F angled catheter
	Confirmation of the proximal obstruction
	Dilatation of the obstruction with a 3 F tapered dilating catheter – this is advanced only 2.5 cm into the tube
	Confirmation of patency (Figures 7.11–7.13)

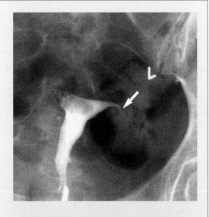

Figure 7.11
Salpingography showing proximal obstruction of the left Fallopian tube (arrow)

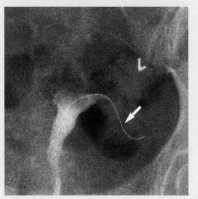

Figure 7.12
Selective canalization of the left tube allowing dilatation of the obstruction

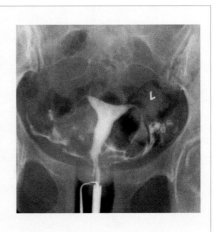

Figure 7.13
Both tubes patent and
showing normal spillage

Outcome

Pregnancy rate:
- 34% with fluoroscopic guidance
- 39% with hysteroscopic guidance

Complications

Pelvic discomfort for approximately 24 h
Tubal perforation (1%)
Ectopic pregnancy (4%)
Infection (0.5%)

7.2 Male Varicocoeles

Presentation

Swelling within the scrotal sac

Predominantly left-sided, although reported incidence of bilateral hydrocoeles varies between 7 and 23%

Subclinical varices thought to make up 44% of all varices

Varicocoeles are found in 37% of subfertile men – various theories have been put forward to explain this; these include testicular dysfunction as a result of increased testicular temperature, hormonal imbalance and reflux metabolites

Investigations

Duplex ultrasound

Sperm evaluation

Venography – to confirm the presence of varicocoeles

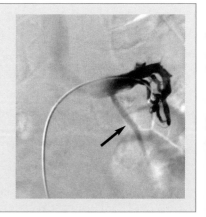

Figure 7.21
Selective left renal vein study showing reflux into the left testicular vein (arrow)

Treatment options

Surgery involving laparoscopic ligation and perioperative spermatic vein sclerosis

Interventional therapy

Diagnosis and treatment can be done at a single sitting

Contraindications

Absolute

Synchronous pathology of the genitourinary tract i.e. carcinoma of the kidney

Relative	Aberrant venous anatomy
Patient preparation	Informed consent
	Appropriate anaesthetic ± sedation
Procedure	Venous access can be achieved by the internal jugular or femoral vein (Figure 7.21)
	Formal venogram of the left renal vein is used to confirm the presence of retrograde flow within the enlarged testicular veins (Figure 7.22)
	The spermatic vein is catheterized and occluded using coils (Figure 7.23) or sclerosant chemicals (alcohol, etc.)

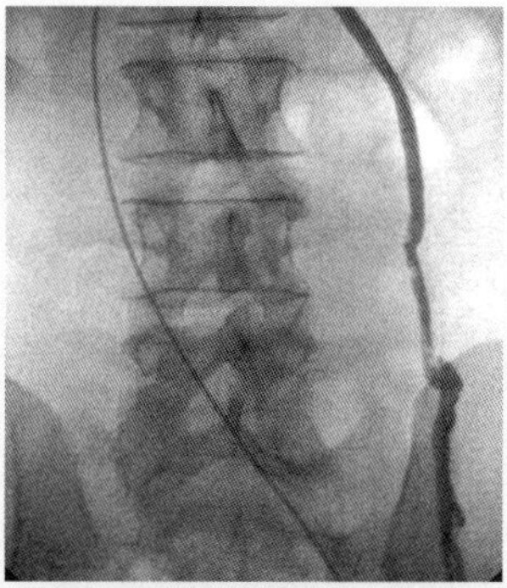

Figure 7.22
Outlined dilated left
testicular vein prior to
embolization

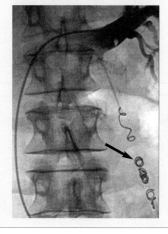

Figure 7.23
Embolization coils
introduced into the left
testicular vein occluding
flow to the left
varicocoele (arrow)

Outcome	Subsequent pregnancy rate is 30–68% (assuming normal partner); this is similar to that following surgical treatment
Complications	Migration of embolic material
	Post-procedural vasovagal episodes
	Testicular phlebitis or infarction (<1%)
	Back pain requiring analgesia (lasting 2-5 days)

TUBAL RECANALIZATION

What is tubal recanalization?

The doctors have discovered that you have a blocked fallopian tube. This may be related to problems of infertility. The obstruction can be relieved by dilatation.

What happens?

In order to see the obstruction within the fallopian tube, the radiologist (X-ray doctor) will introduce a tube (catheter) into your fallopian tube, through the vagina and womb. You will have an X-ray tube over your abdomen so that the radiologist can see the dye. If a narrowing is seen he will attempt to widen the tube.

How long will it take?

The procedure usually takes about 1 h, although you can expect to be in the department for about 2 h.

Is it painful?

There is some discomfort with the internal examination and period-like pains when the dye is introduced and the narrowing of the tube expanded. If necessary you can have a sedative/pain killing injection via a vein in your hand.

Afterwards

You will return to the ward for observation. Your doctor will discuss the results of the procedure with you.

VARICOCOELE EMBOLIZATION

What is varicocoele embolization?

The doctors have discovered that you have enlarged veins within your scrotum that need to be deliberately blocked off.

What happens?

In order to see the enlarged veins within the scrotum, the radiologist (X-ray doctor) will introduce a tube (catheter) into your scrotum, via the groin. You will have an X-ray tube over your abdomen so that the radiologist can see the dye. Once identified the dilated veins will be blocked with metal coils.

How long will it take?

The procedure usually takes about 1 h, although you can expect to be in the department for about 2 h.

Is it painful?

There is some minor discomfort with the blocking of the veins. If necessary you can have a sedative/pain killing injection via a vein in your hand.

Afterwards

You will return to the ward for observation. Your doctor will discuss the results of the procedure with you.

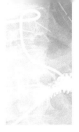

APPENDIX

The Seldinger technique

This technique is used in modified forms to gain safe access to any vessel, cavity (abscess) or lumen of any organ (kidney, gall bladder)

Figure 1.1
The vessel is transfixed using a two-part needle. With a one-part needle a single wall puncture is performed

Figure 1.2
The inner needle is removed and the trochar withdrawn into the vessel lumen until good backflow is achieved

Figure 1.3
A guidewire is introduced into the vessel, through the trochar

Figure 1.4
The trochar is removed and a catheter advanced over the guidewire.
Angioplasty can be performed via the catheter

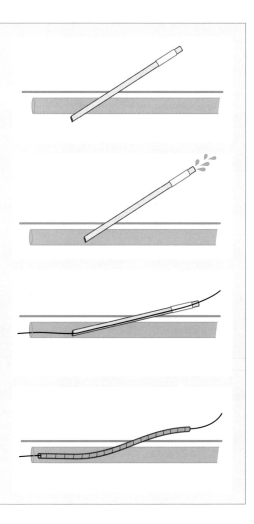

INDEX